StyleItaliano

ONE-DAY VENEERING

Yearbook 2023

Books Editor in Chief: Paola Sammaritano, Edra S.p.A.
Books Project Manager: Sandra A. Calarota, Edra S.p.A.
Paper, Printing and Binding Manager: Paolo Ficicchia, Edra S.p.A.
Cover: Ursula Giusti, Edra S.p.A.
Layout: Barbara Rastelli

ISBN: 9781962679992
eISBN: 9781962679329

edra
PUBLISHING

Edra Publishing US LLC
3309 Northlake Boulevard,
Suite 203,
Palm Beach Gardens,
FL 33403
EIN: 844113980
info@edrapublishing.com
www.edrapublishing.com

Printed in July 2024 by "Erregiemme printing" S.r.l.

StyleItaliano

ONE-DAY VENEERING

Yearbook 2023

STYLE ITALIANO Certified SHADE GUIDES

edra PUBLISHING

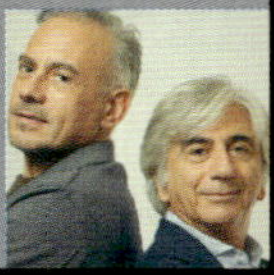

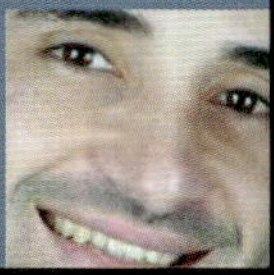

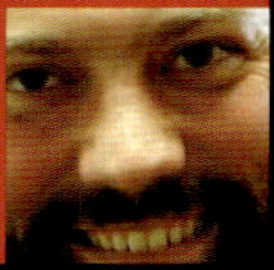

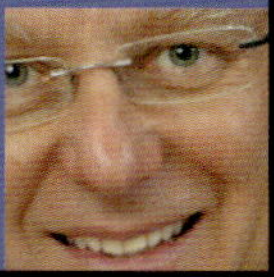

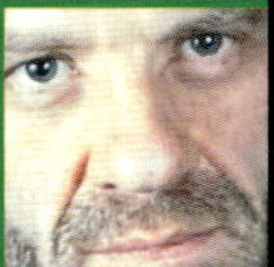

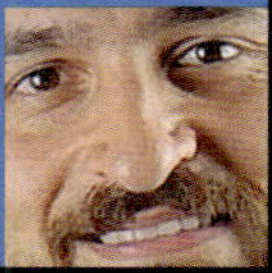

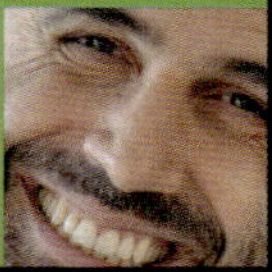

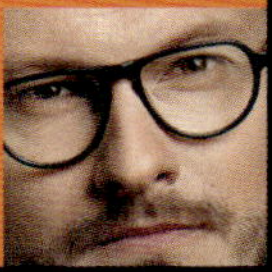

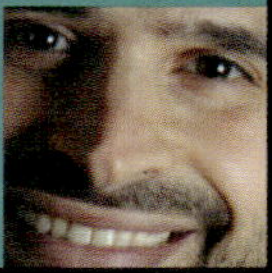

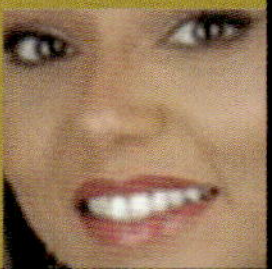

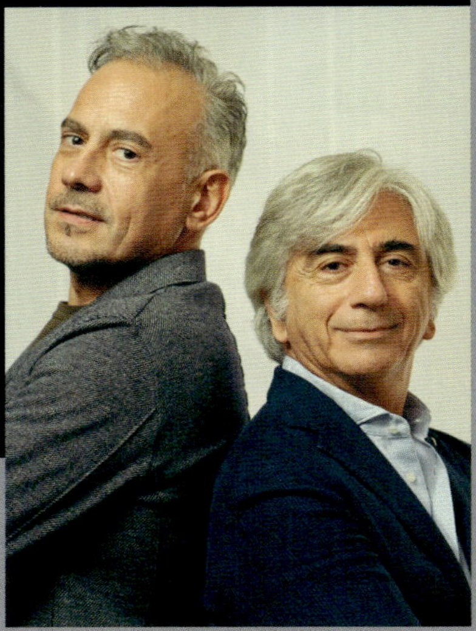

WALTER DEVOTO, ANGELO PUTIGNANO

Italy

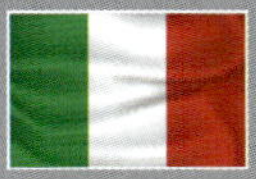

WALTER DEVOTO

Graduated cum laude in Dentistry and Dental Prosthetics from the University of Genoa. He has held teaching and demonstrator positions over the years at several universities worldwide in the subjects of Pedodontics, Reconstructive Dentistry, Laser and Dental Aesthetics.
Currently Visiting Professor at the Postgraduate Course in Aesthetic Reconstructive Dentistry, Universitè de la Mediterranèe, Marseille, and at the International University of Catalonia, Barcelona, on the Master's Course in Aesthetic Dentistry.
Adjunct Professor at the Polytechnic University of the Marches, Ancona.

Particularly interested in aesthetic conservative restoration, he is the author and co-author of 85 publications in specialized international journals and 8 books published in 10 languages.
He has organized more than 200 courses in the StyleItaliano Course Center in Italy with 4000 participants and given 600 presentations in 80 countries worldwide on the subject. Founder of the Styleitaliano.org group, an educational community recognized worldwide with nearly 500,000 followers, he has developed innovative techniques, tools and materials in cooperation with multiple companies in the field.

Member of the Academy of Operative Dentistry since 1996. Active member of the Italian Academy of Conservative Dentistry since 1998. Active member of the European Academy of Aesthetic Dentistry since 2002. Founder of the Italian Academy of Esthetic Dentistry. Founder of StyleItaliano, Styleitaliano.org.
He practices in Sestri Levante, Chiavari and in Santa Margherita Ligure (Genoa), and collaborates with prestigious aesthetic dental practices throughout Europe.

PREFACE

ANGELO PUTIGNANO

Graduated from the Faculty of Medicine of the Polytechnic University of the Marches, where he also specialized in the School of Dentistry. Since the beginning of his career he has lectured internationally on adhesive and aesthetic restorations.

He is a full professor of Restorative Dentistry at the Faculty of Dentistry of the Polytechnic University of Marches and is the head of the Department of Operative Dentistry and Endodontics at the same university. He has also collaborated with the University of Barcelona and the University of Marseille as a visiting professor. He received the Certificate of Excellence as a dental lecturer and educator at Tufts University (Boston).

He has authored numerous clinical and research articles on aesthetics and adhesive dentistry and is an internationally renowned speaker on these topics, with more than 200 published articles. He recently became dean of the School of Dentistry at the Polytechnic University of the Marches. Over the years he has been active in important dental societies: he was President of the Italian Society of Conservative Dentistry (SIDOC), Founding Member of the Italian Academy of Esthetic Dentistry (IAED) and Active Member of the European Academy of Esthetic Dentistry (EAED). He is co-author of the books *Adhesive Dentistry: the Key to Success* (Quintessence International, 2007), *Indirect Conservative Restoration of Posterior Teeth* (UTET, 2008), *Layers 2* (Quintessence International, 2022).

He is co-founder of the dental group StyleItaliano, which has nearly 500,000 followers worldwide and offers ideas that help dentists deal with daily challenges in their dental practice.

Anterior tooth restoration is "the signature" of the dentist. The patient has increasingly demanding expectations, thanks also to competition, global information and social media. They want high-performance, non-invasive restorations that satisfy their aesthetic identity, all in just a few appointments and with affordable costs. The challenge is certainly curious and we at StyleItaliano have accepted it: in this volume we have collected different solutions from our followers from all over the world, to meet the aesthetic needs of our patients in just one appointment, with direct and indirect techniques, taking full advantage of digital technology.

This is StyleItaliano: giving voice and visibility to the passion for our work.

Happy reading!
Angelo & Walter

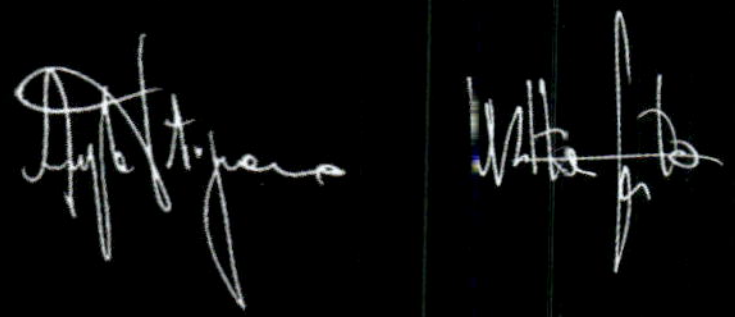

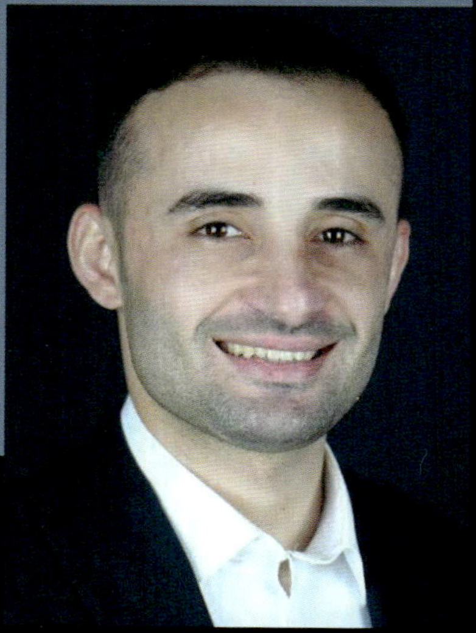

OSAMA SHAALAN

Palestine

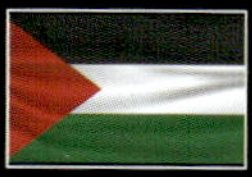

Osama Shaalan was born in Palestine. He graduated with honors in Dentistry in 2013 from the University of Sinai.
He is the director of several courses in Palestine on direct composite restoration techniques.
He is the inventor of the posterior replica instrument for direct posterior composite modeling and occlusal shaping of posterior teeth.
He is a certified member of the European Society of Cosmetic Dentistry (ESCD), which awarded him as the youngest and most promising dentist on the 20th anniversary of the ESCD in 2023.
He is the first Gold Member of StyleItaliano in the Middle East.
He is an international lecturer for aesthetic and restorative dentistry.
He is the author of numerous articles and publications in the field of dental aesthetics.
He is a key opinion leader for many international dental companies. Dr. Shaalan has maintained his clinical practice in aesthetics and restorative dentistry in his private clinic in Palestine.

INTRODUCTION: ONE-DAY VENEERING

They say the smile is a curve that sets everything straight.
A beautiful smile means a happy life because this is particularly important to gain confidence and for successful daily relationships. How do you make the patients happy? The goal of any dental treatment is to reach patient satisfaction and to make them happy. The most common problem when patients come to the dental office is that the majority of them cannot afford expensive treatments. Another is when dentists offer them invasive options or over-treatment that affect the quality of their smile. So, it is a must to respect the patient needs by providing them with the treatment they deserve using minimally invasive options and when deciding the treatment plan there should an integration between biology, structure, function, and aesthetics[1].
Today this has become real with the introduction of new techniques, materials, and instruments everything is simplified in terms of the procedure and the overall time. This book will discuss the StyleItaliano techniques for using anterior direct composite restorations for those who are looking for a more affordable and minimally invasive smile makeover in a single visit.

THE CONCEPT OF ONE-DAY VENEERING

With an emphasis on the emergence of direct composite veneers, the coming years look to be historic for smile makeovers in the rapidly changing field of dentistry. Direct composite veneers have gained an important role in dental clinical applications following recently developed materials and techniques in adhesive and restorative dentistry and having the ability to change the patient's smile in one visit nowadays is considered a miracle, because we are not only changing their smile but also their life[2]. This choice creates new possibilities for minimally invasive dentistry as the tooth shape, position, and color can be altered without loss of tooth substance in one visit[3] (📷 1, 2).

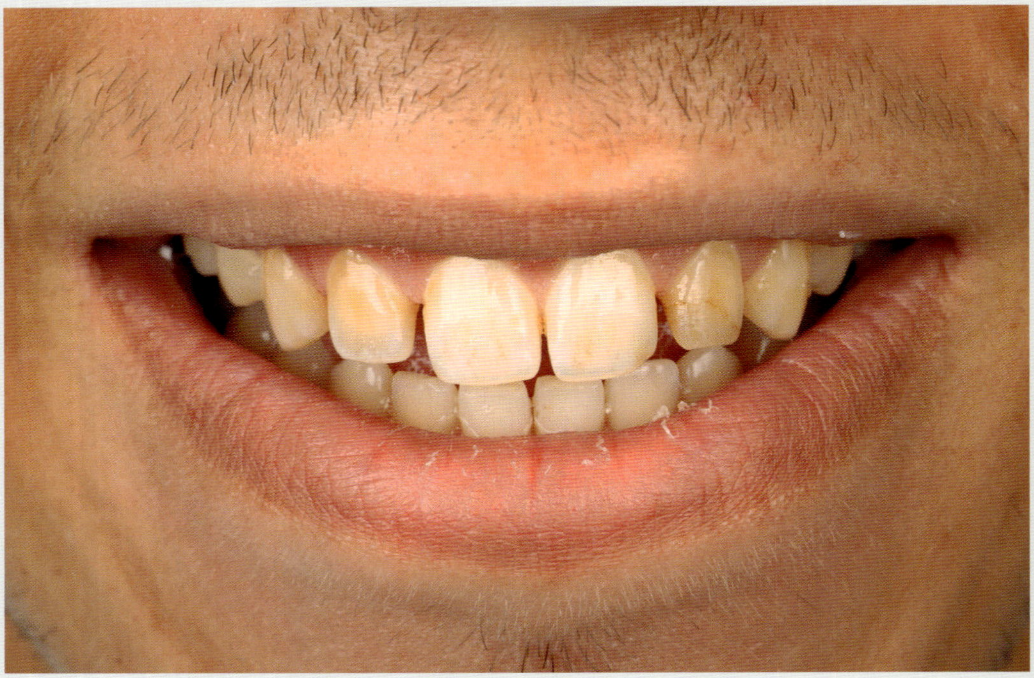

Figure 1 Before the intervention.

Advantages of one-day veneering

- A single visit is a life-changing procedure as compared to other treatments like porcelain veneers which need at least three visits.
- Minimally invasive: direct composite veneers are a conservative alternative because they don't require much tooth preparation.
- Many issues such as discolorations, chipping, gaps, and misalignments can be solved in one visit.
- Natural appearance: the composite material creates a flawless, lifelike smile by simulating the appearance of natural teeth in a short time.
- Cost-effective as compared to other dental aesthetic treatments[4-6].

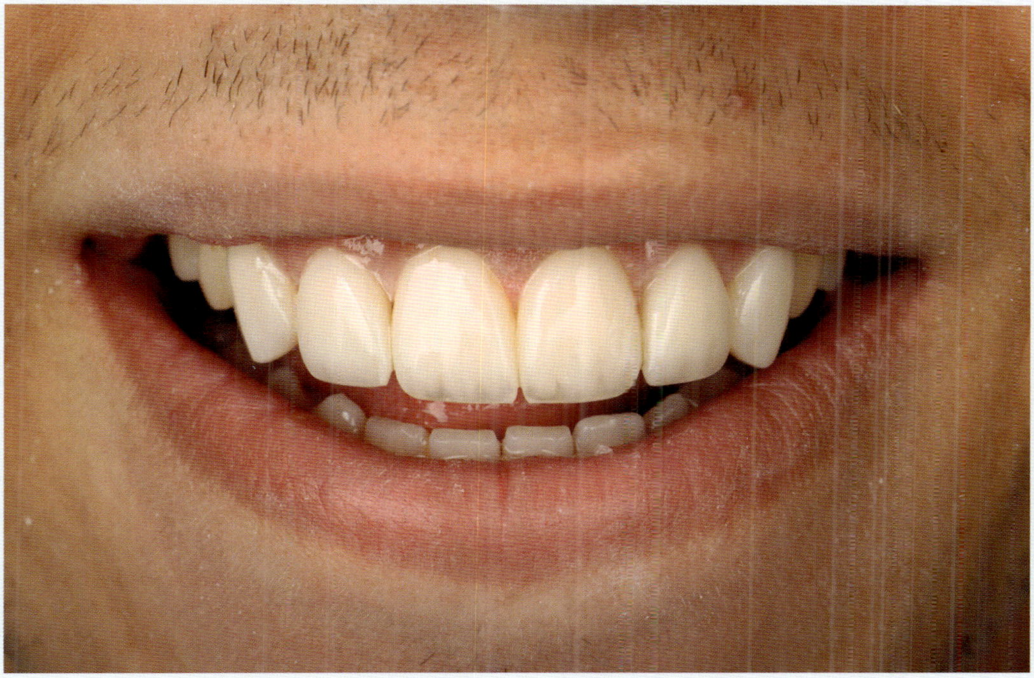

Figure 2 After a smile makeover with a direct composite.

Simplified layering technique

There are four recipes for doing a direct composite veneer for color enhancement or masking discoloration and shape modifications (📷 3, 4).

1. Using only one dentin shade for the entire labial surface, simple and fast, can be used in situations for patients with either worn incisal edges or just from day-to-day habits, has thin enamel due to age; we do not suggest the use of an enamel shade. Providing the shade and shape are often correct; we only need to use one body shade with CompoSite (Optident-UK), simplifying the technique[7].
2. Using one dentin for the labial surface and proximal walls with enamel shade only on the incisal third. Simple, fast, and natural (the most used). In instances where a younger patient needs a little more brightness, the Si E shade (Enamel) is the perfect option, as it takes up the color of the body material for a natural appearance.
3. Using one dentin and enamel for the entire labial surface is more natural. Still, one needs to be careful to control the thickness of the whole enamel on the labial surface, not exceeding 0.5 mm[8].
4. In case of severe discoloration or very dark teeth, we use a masking agent in addition to dentin and enamel. This technique is called the camouflage technique that covers the discoloration with a light foundation[7].

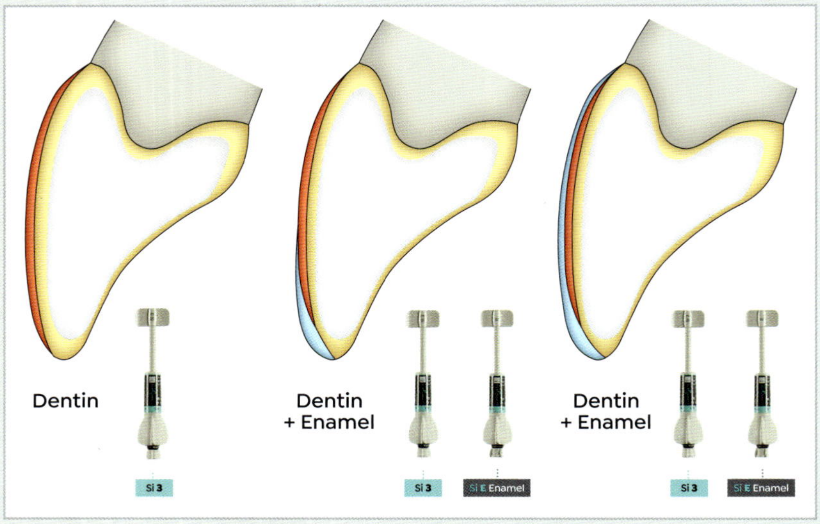

Figure 3 Layering recipes: 1: one dentin shade;
2 shades: one dentin and only enamel at the incisal edge;
2 shades: one dentin and one enamel covering the entire surface.

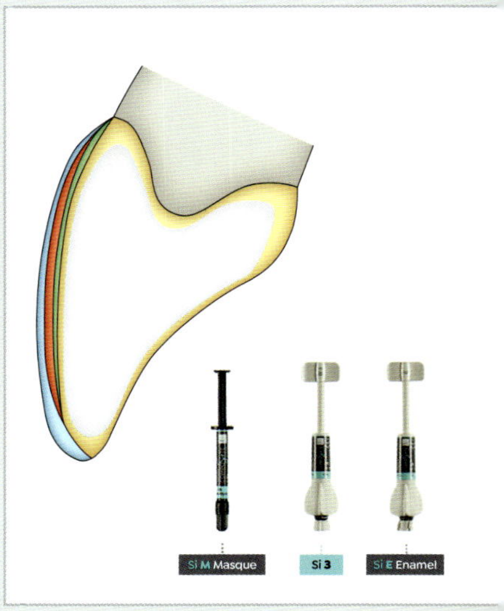

Figure 4 Severe discoloration recipe using a masking agent in addition to dentin and enamel.

Clinical case

A 25-year-old young woman comes to the clinic after having orthodontic treatment and she wants to have a beautiful and confident smile (5, 6b). In the retracted view there are multiple old composite restorations with disharmony between the teeth's shape between the right and the left (6b,c). Treatment planning (based on the discussion with the patient), resin composite veneering with minimal tooth preparation was planned (6a). In agreement with the patient's wishes, we decided to do composite veneers as a minimally invasive approach to modify both the color and shape of the upper anterior teeth with direct composite veneering from the 4-4 as appeared from the full smile and to correct the flat smile curve.

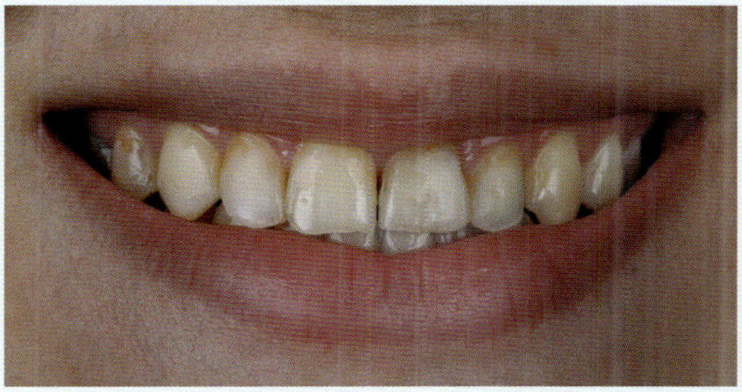

Figure 5 Initial situation, full smile.

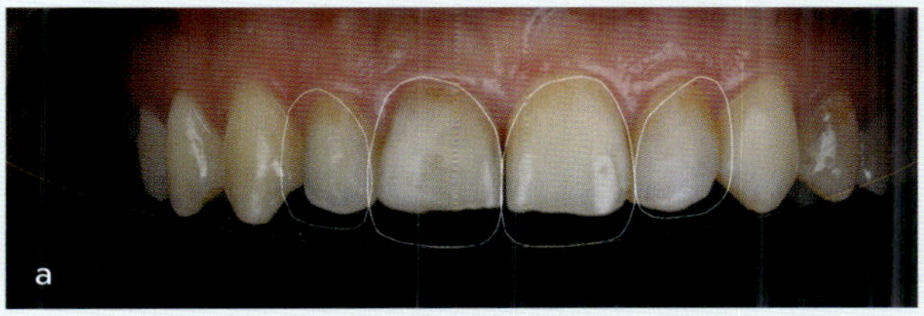

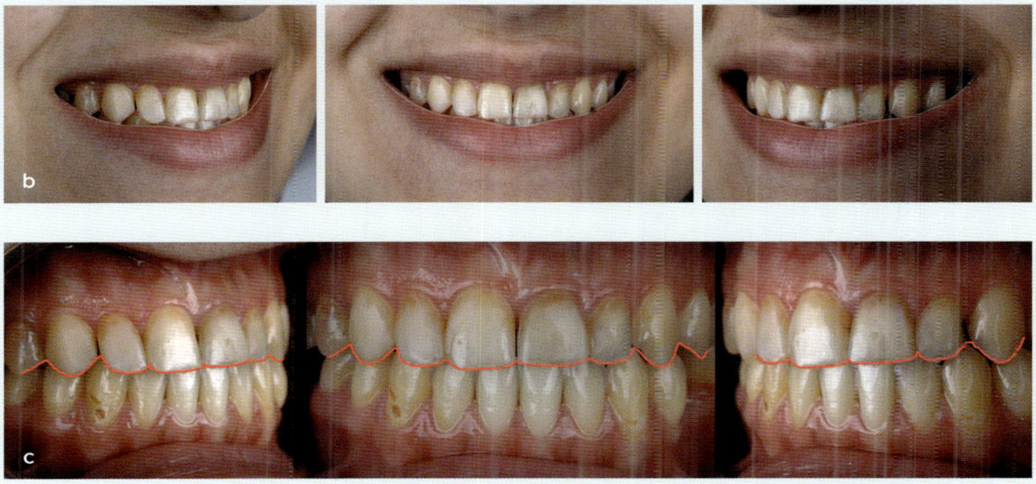

Figure 6 Black contrast - treatment plan.
(a) Increase the length of 4 anterior to correspond that to the curve of the smile and lower lip.
(b) Enhance the color of the teeth. Correction of the shape symmetry between the right and left side.
(c) Correction of the smile curve and incisal embrasure

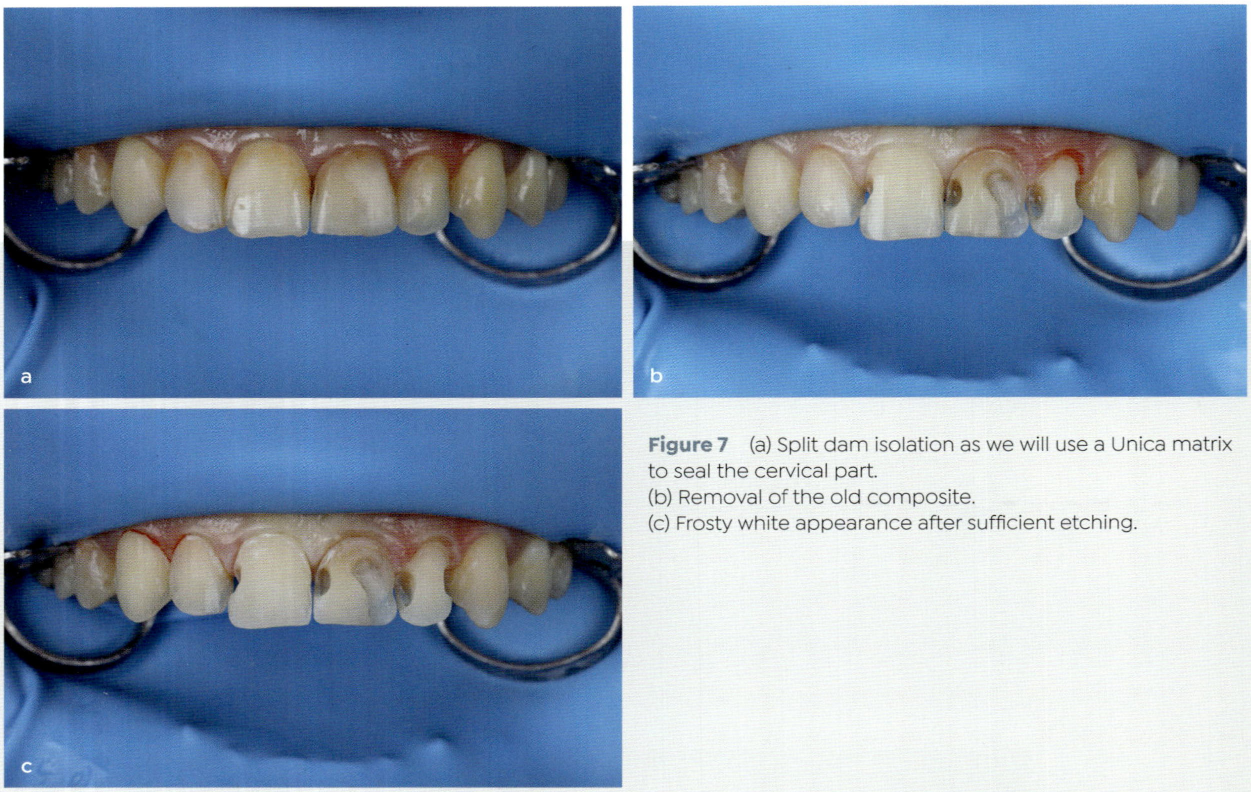

Figure 7 (a) Split dam isolation as we will use a Unica matrix to seal the cervical part.
(b) Removal of the old composite.
(c) Frosty white appearance after sufficient etching.

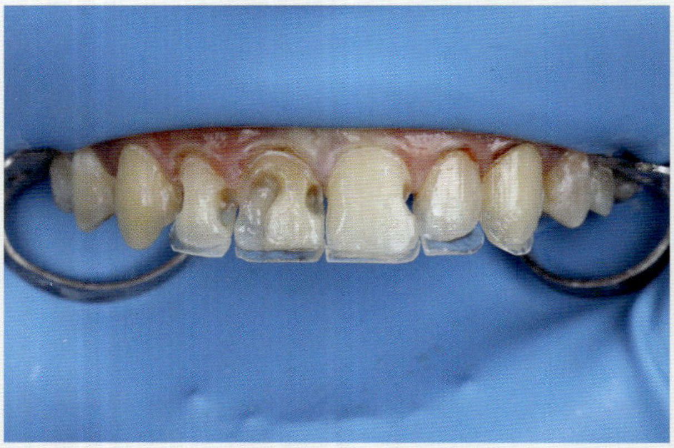

Figure 8 Freehand construction of palatal shell using mylar strip supported palatally by a finger as this will be done in a single visit. A little pre-finishing of the palatal shell before proceeding to the next step.

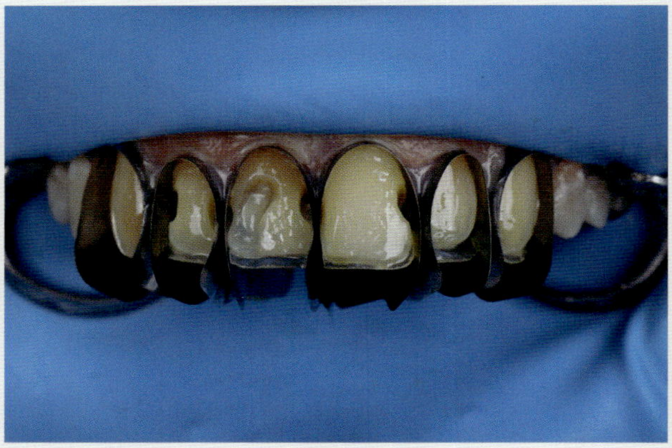

Figure 9 Multiple Unica matrix in action (build, support, and predict) – Unica anterior (Polydentia – Switzerland). A Unica matrix that can wrap around the tooth in all directions enabling the practitioner to build the proximal and cervical in one shot. There are two types of Unica matrix: regular for large teeth like upper central and canine and mini-deep for small teeth like upper lateral and lower teeth[7].

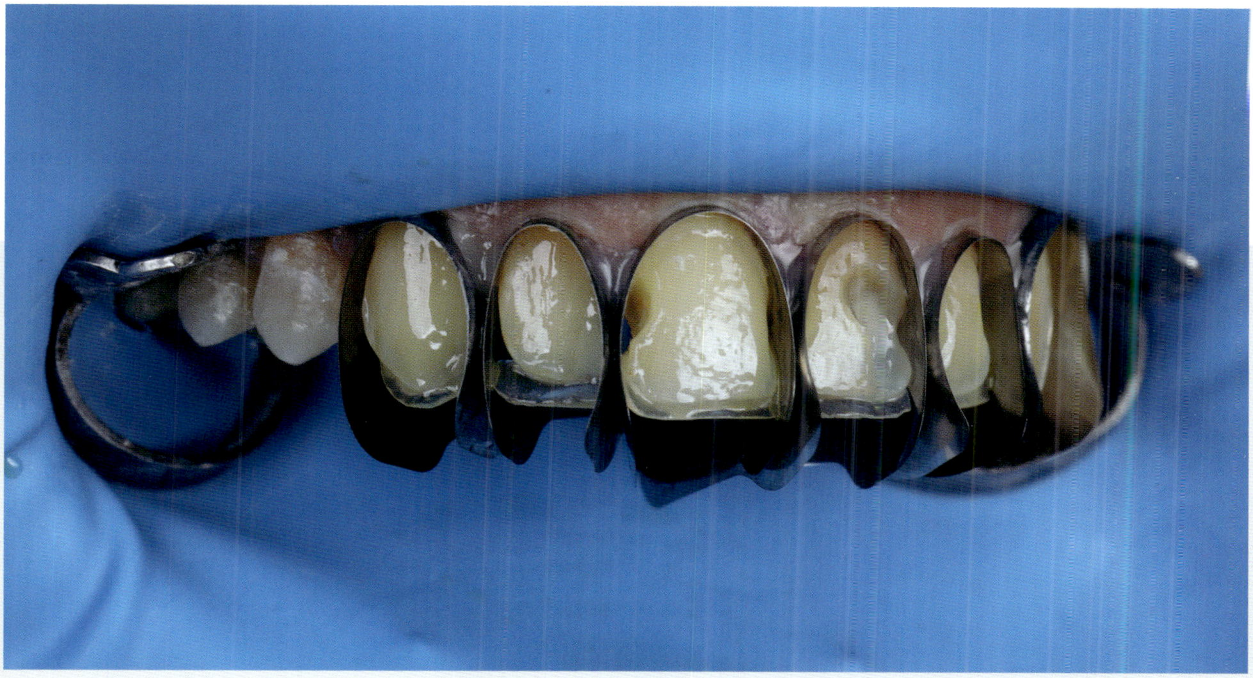

Figure 10 Side view Unica matrix that can predict and visualize the outer shape and contour of the final restorations.

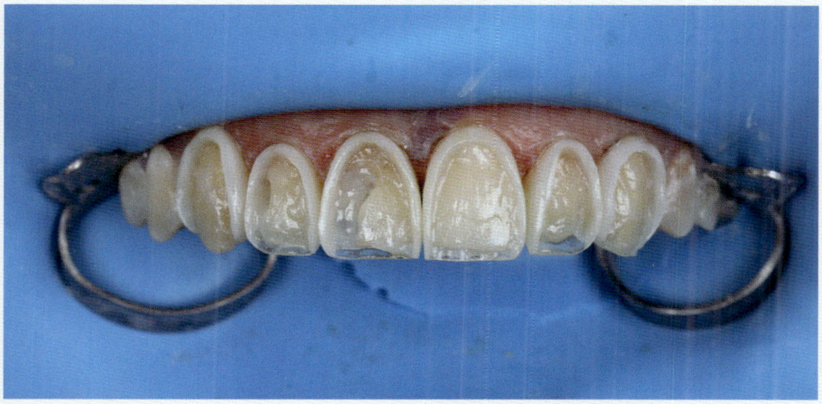

Figure 11 A frame is produced when building the proximal walls and cervical from the Unica matrix, which helps predict the restorations' final shape, control the amount of composite material during layering, and subsequently decrease the time of the finishing and polishing.

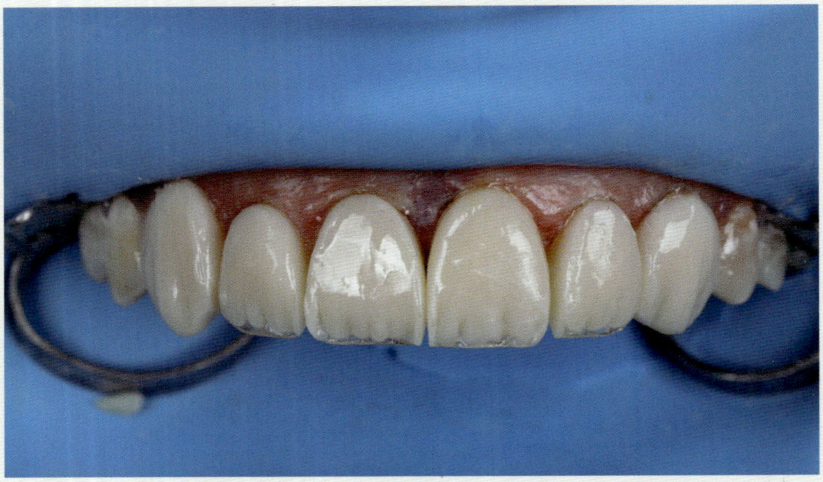

Figure 12 Layering the veneering material which is the same dentine shade of the proximal walls.

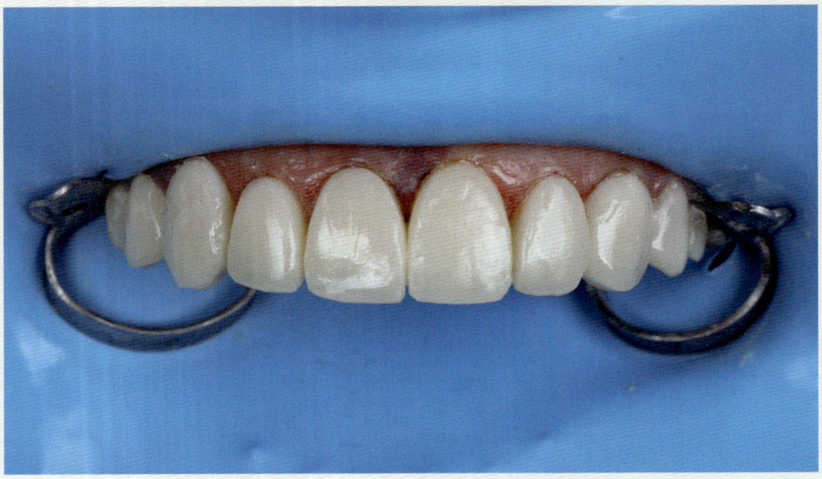

Figure 13 Layering the final enamel layer up to incisal 1/3.

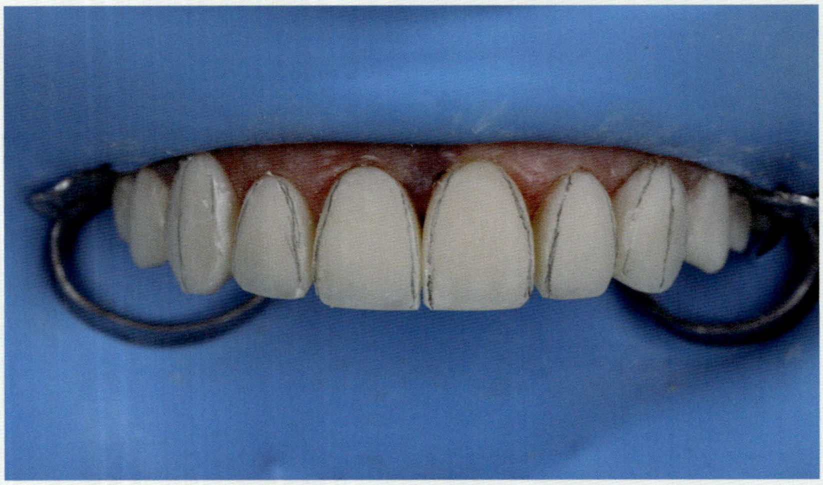

Figure 14 Finishing process.

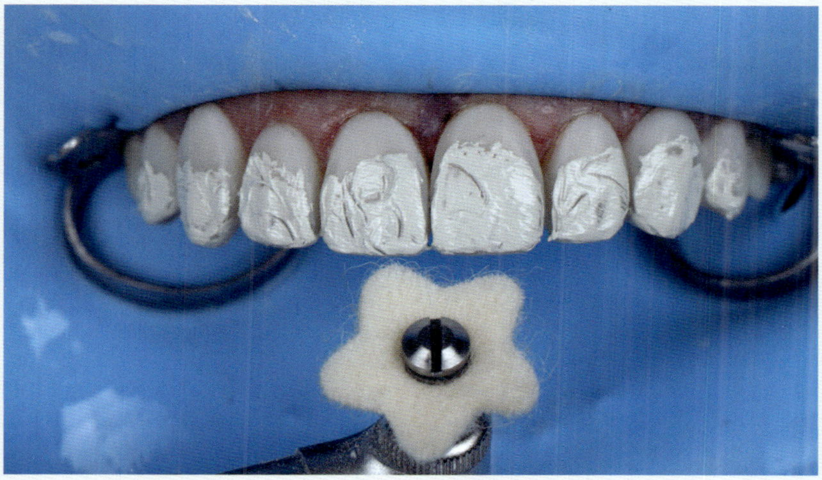

Figure 15 Final polishing step using Lucida polishing from Diashine.

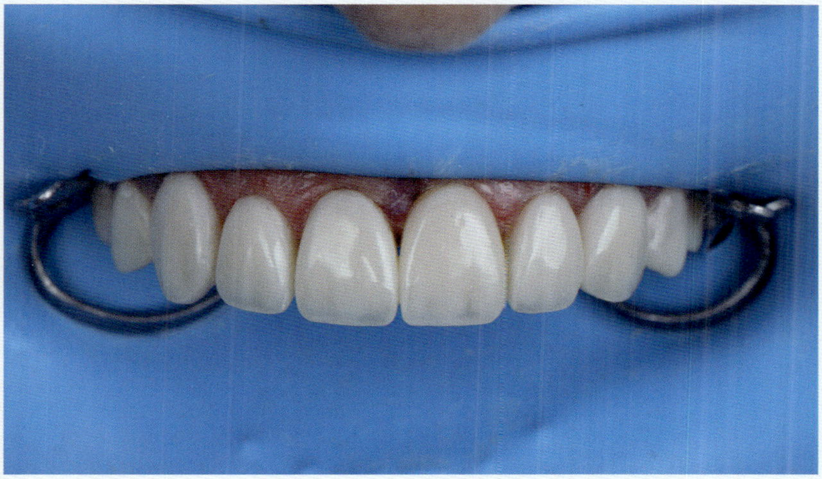

Figure 16 Immediately after with surface gloss.

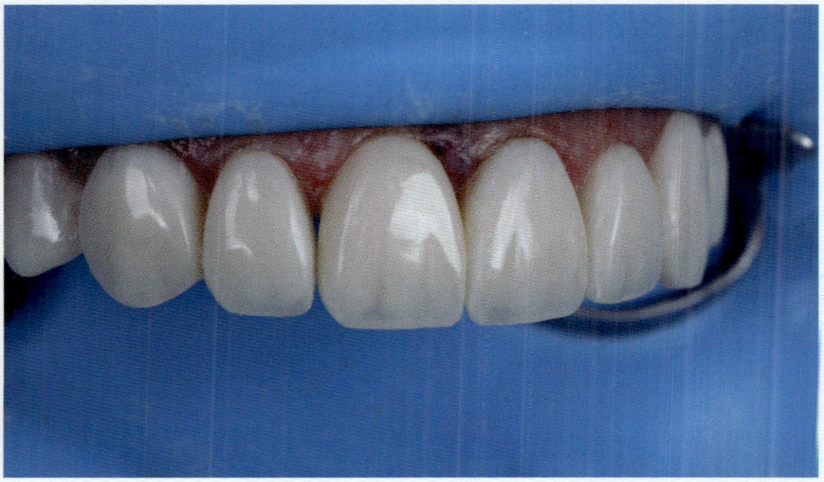

Figure 17 Side view.

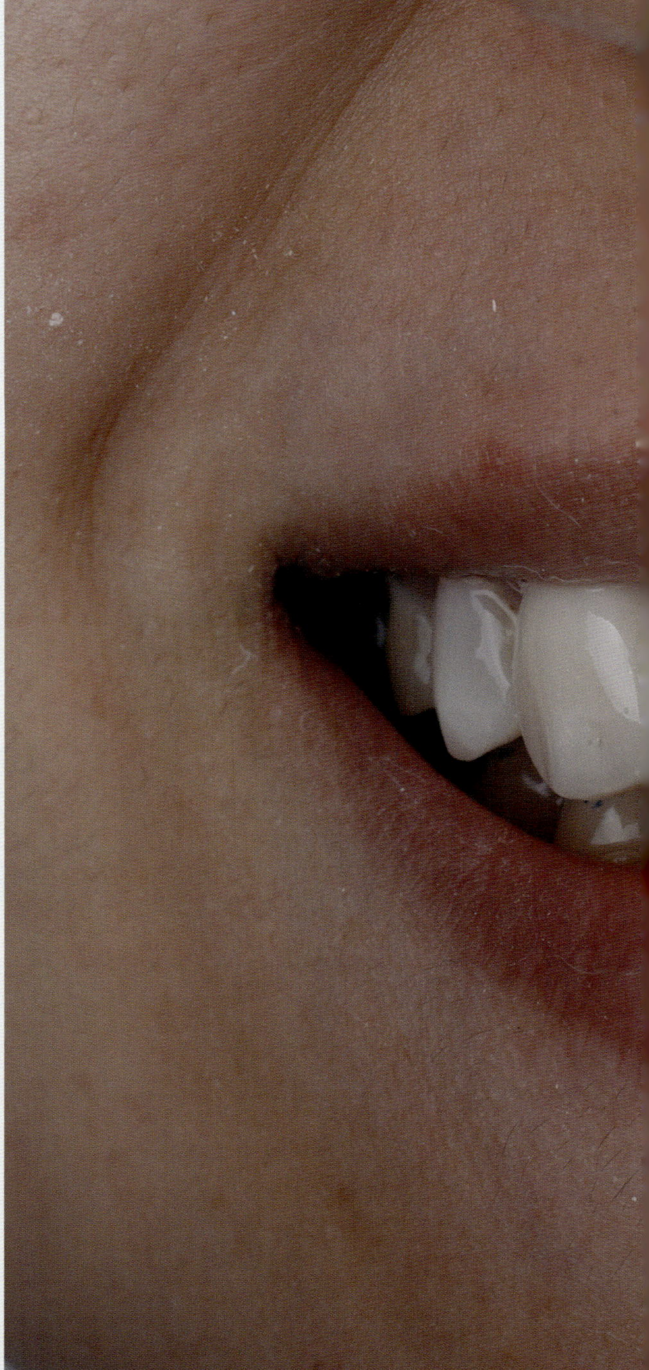

Figure 18 Final aesthetic result.

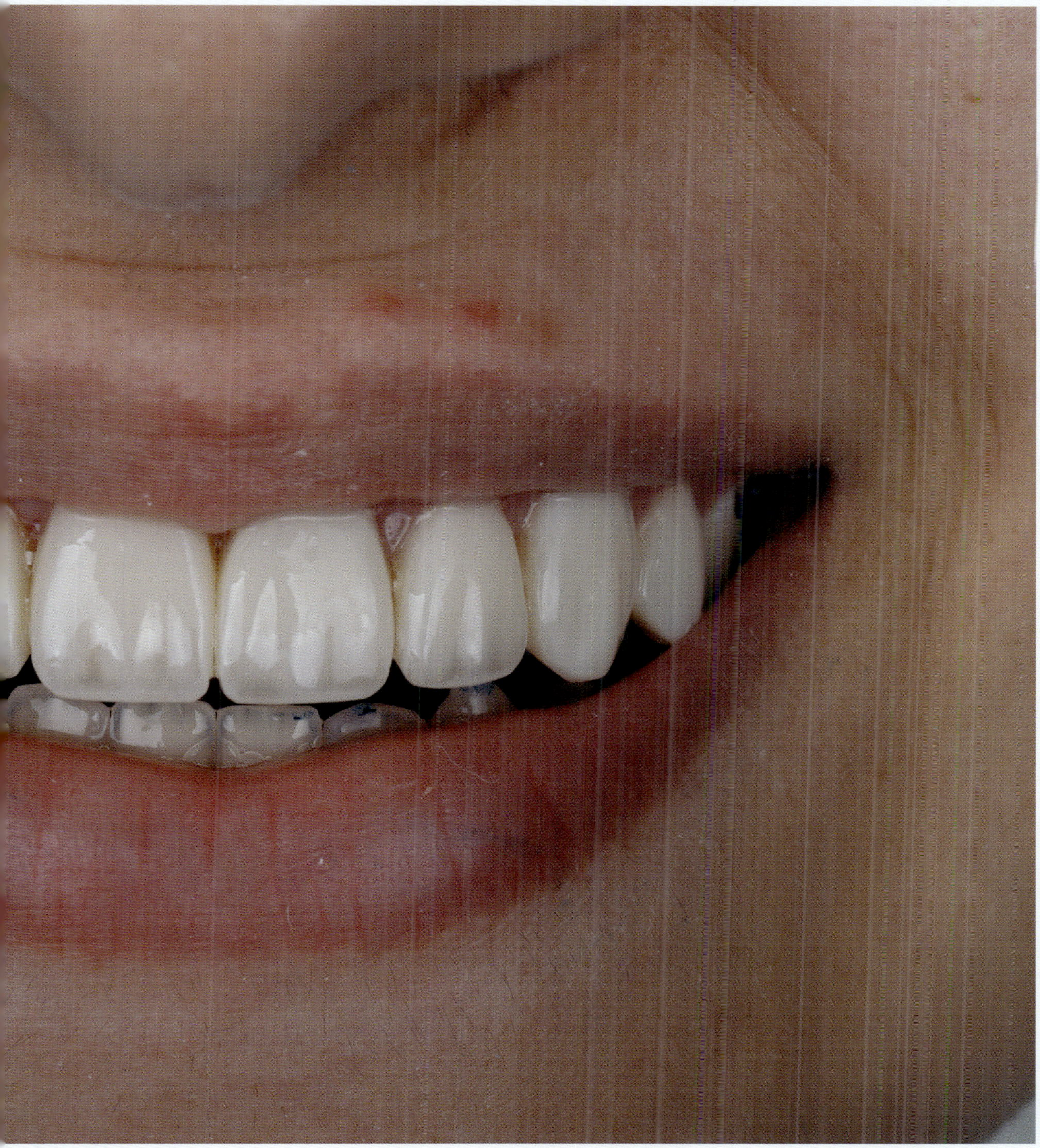

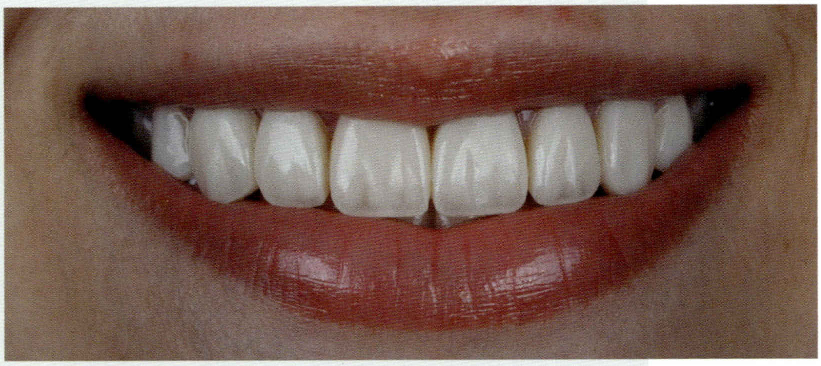

Figure 19 One-week follow-up.

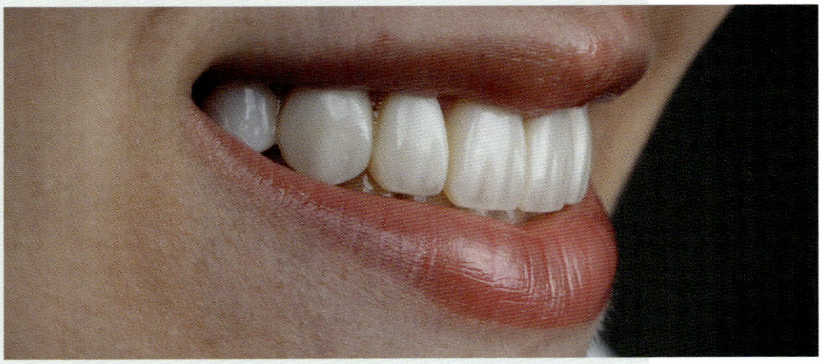

Figure 20 Side view.

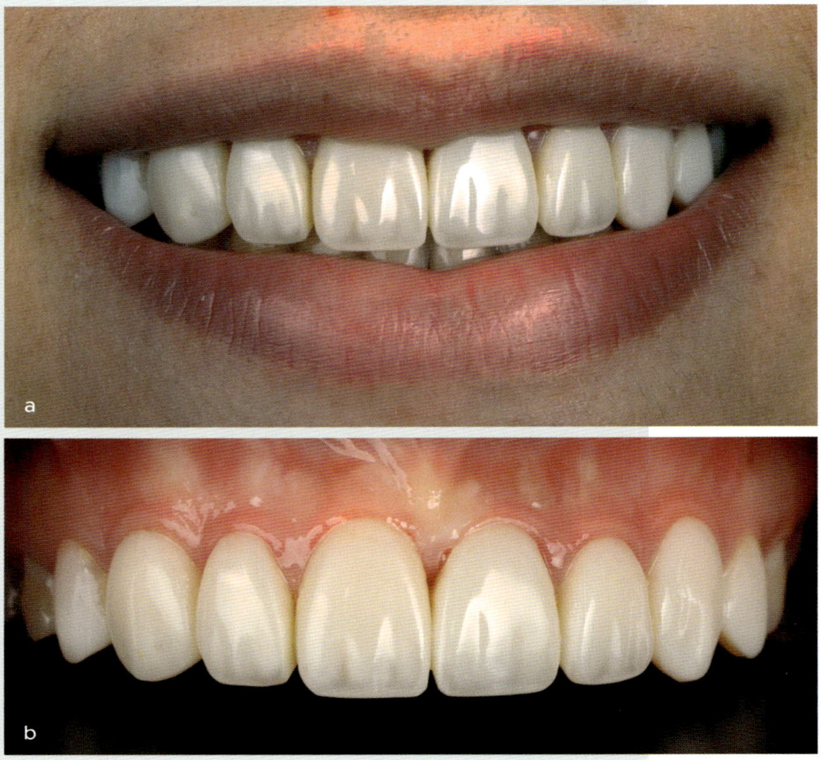

Figure 21 One-year follow-up.

CONCLUSION

Direct composite veneers are a contemporary and cost-effective option for people thinking about changing their smiles, in a minimally invasive way and this can be done in just one visit, reducing the time on both the patient and the practitioner.

REFERENCES

1. Spear FM, Kokich VG. A multidisciplinary approach to esthetic dentistry. *Dent Clin North Am.* 2007;51(2):487-505.
2. Korkut B. Smile makeover with direct composite veneers: A two-year follow-up report. *J Dent Res Dent Clin Dent Prospects.* 2018;12(2):146-151.
3. Desai H, Stewart CA, Finer Y. Minimally Invasive Therapies for the Management of Dental Caries-A Literature Review. *Dent J (Basel).* 2021;9(12):147.
4. Araujo E, Perdigão J. Anterior Veneer Restorations - An Evidence-based Minimal-Intervention Perspective. *J Aches Dent.* 2021;23(2):91-110.
5. Lundergan WP, Lyon L. Research on hand dexterity and the practice of dentistry: reality and myth. *J Am Coll Dent.* 2007;74(3):15-6.
6. Re D, Augusti G, Amato M, Riva G, Augusti D. Esthetic rehabilitation of anterior teeth with laminates composite veneers. *Case Rep Dent.* 2014; 2014:849273.
7. StyleItaliano. *Yearbook 2022.* Edra Publishing 2023.
8. Manauta J, Salat A, Devoto W, Putignano A. *Layers 2. Direct Composites: The StyleItaliano Clinical Secrets.* Quintessence Publishing, 2022.

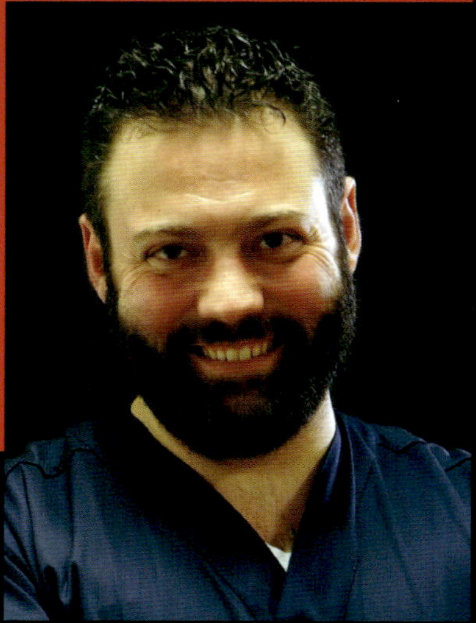

GIULIO PAVOLUCCI

Italy

Giulio Pavolucci was born in Siena in 1984. After graduating from high school, he graduated with honors in Dentistry and Dental Prosthetics from the University of Siena in July 2009. At the same university he was Adjunct Professor of Restorative Dentistry in the academic year 2010/2011 and from 2014 to the present, and Lecturer on the Master's Degree Course in Conservative and Endodontics by Prof. Grandini from 2010 to the present. He is an honorary member of the StyleItaliano group and an active member of SIDOC (Italian Society of Conservative Dentistry).

A speaker in courses and congresses, he carries out clinical practice focusing mainly on direct and indirect aesthetic restorative.

LAST BUT NOT LEAST: CONTOURING, FINISHING AND POLISHING

When it comes to the end of a complex mucogingival surgery, the suture phase is by no means marginal and can strongly influence the final result. This is also the case with direct aesthetic restorations: it is true that the central phase is the layering of the material, but the finishing and polishing procedures are equally fundamental. In the age-old question of the predominance of color or shape, there is no real winner: both color and achromatic characteristics are essential to achieve a good result. However, the importance of shape and surface texture must be recognized, especially when considering the point of view of the ordinary observer.
In a high-magnification photograph it will be easy to distinguish even small color errors, but when observing with the naked eye, correct morphology and natural-looking surface texture can compensate for some color errors, making the result pleasing to the eye of the observer.
Let's not forget that it is precisely the shapes of the macro- and micro-anatomy that regulate the way light is reflected. When it comes to the finishing stage, therefore, it is advisable to keep your concentration high, taking your time to perform all the steps to the best of your ability. In cases where there are strong doubts about the color component (and therefore a high risk of having to remove the composite at the next appointment to correct the error), or in the absence of time, it is possible to postpone the micro-anatomy definition phase to the following session. At first, it is essential to verify that everything is working from a functional point of view and that the restoration is respecting the soft tissue: the rest can also be postponed.

CONTOURING

This step is needed to define the primary anatomy of the tooth. The parameters to be considered are:

- contour
- shape
- orientation
- direction and position of the transition lines.

It is obvious that in partial restorations, such as Class III and IV, contouring is limited to the homologation of the restoration to the contour of the natural tooth. In the case of complete veneers, on the other hand, there is the possibility of intervening by modifying all parameters. These changes, which begin in the project phase (wax-up

Figure 1 Example of mass layering in a central incisor. Definition of contour (a,b), dentin masses (c,d), incisal characterization (e), outline of transition lines (f), completion of buccal surface (g,h).

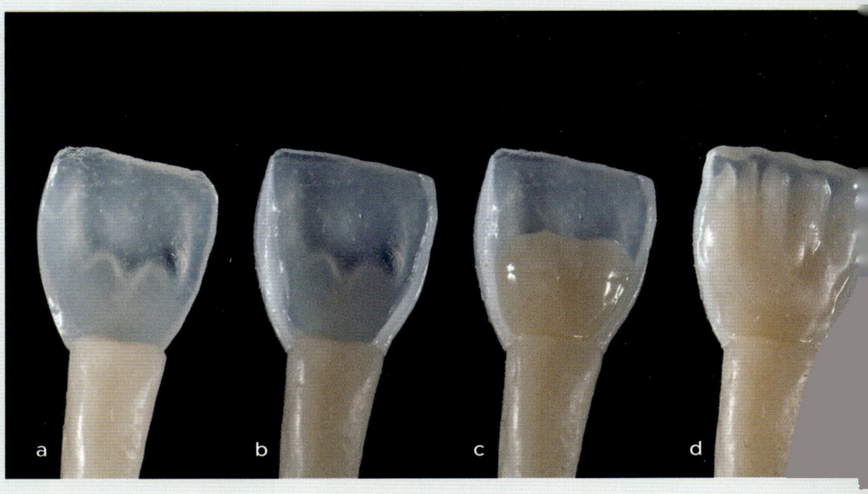

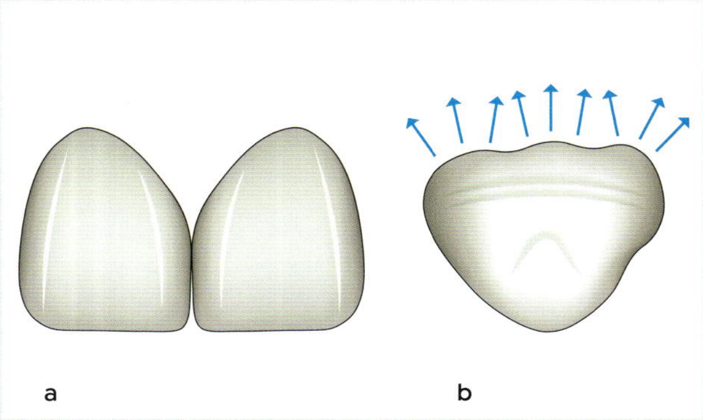

Figure 2 Starting situation with transition lines (a), and iconographic representation of reflected light (b).

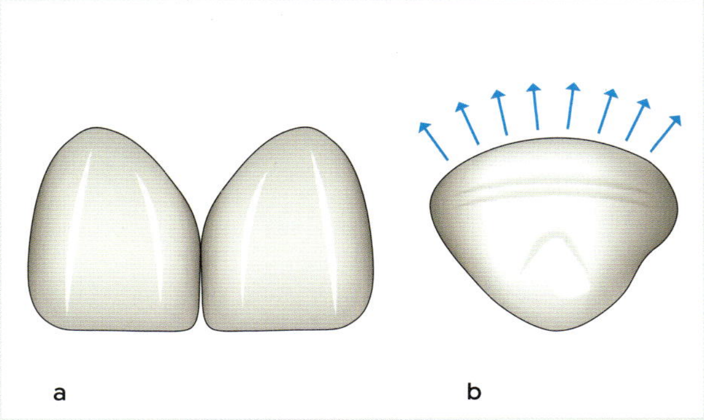

Figure 3 Shift of transition lines towards the center (a) and iconographic representation of reflected light (b).

and mock-up), are draft by composite layering (📷 1), and then defined through the contouring phase.

In some cases, we can create true optical illusions by modifying, for example, the transition lines (📷 2): moving them towards the center of the buccal surface will give an illusion of elongation of the tooth, which will appear slimmer (📷 3).

This effect is very important, for example, when closing diastemas with an additive technique. It can happen that diastematous teeth have a good dimensional harmony between height and width, and that the closure of the spaces results in a squat and less pleasant appearance. Within certain limits, modifying the transition lines can be of great help, especially if there is no possibility of modifying the length of the tooth to compensate for the new width.

Conversely, shifting the transition lines towards the outer edges can give the illusion of wider teeth (📷 4).

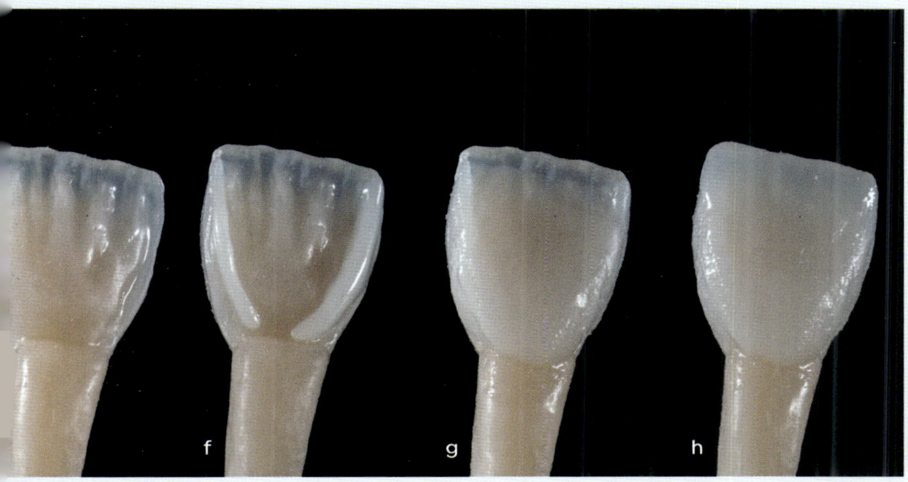

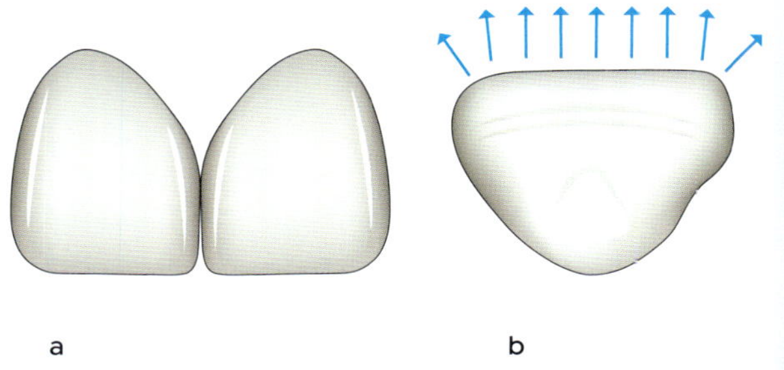

Figure 4 Shifting transition lines to the edges (a) and iconographic representation of reflected light (b).

Basic form

It is a good idea to define the basic form as early as possible during the application of the material, correcting any errors immediately **(📷 5)**. The use of silicone keys based on a wax-up is of great help.

If macroscopic corrections of the shape of the incisal edge are necessary at the end of modelling, a diamond disc can be used **(📷 6)**.

Any characterization of the shape of the incisal edge can be carried out using a flame bur, creating more or less accentuated irregularities as required **(📷 7)**.

The incisal edges can also be defined at this stage. Often underestimated, these elements are very important for the final result and also influence the "personality" of the teeth. Sharp edges, often associated with a sharp, straight incisal edge, denote a certain aggressiveness **(📷 8a,b)**. Conversely, rounding the edges and, especially in lateral incisors, making the incisal margin more sinuous, leads to a more delicate smile **(📷 8c,d)**.

Figure 5 After execution of the palatal wall, inaccuracies are noted in the incisal edge (a), which are immediately corrected (b).

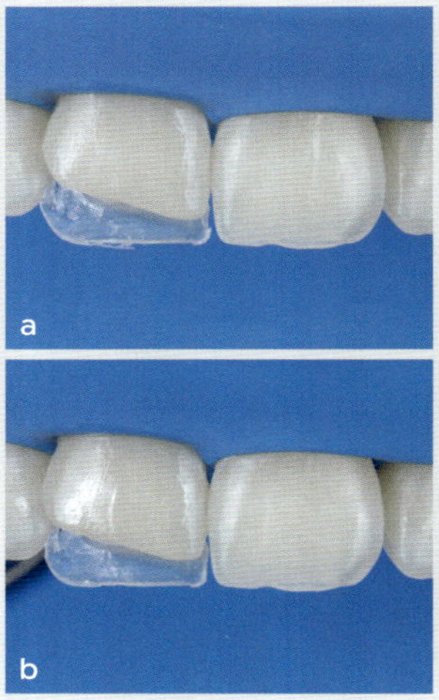

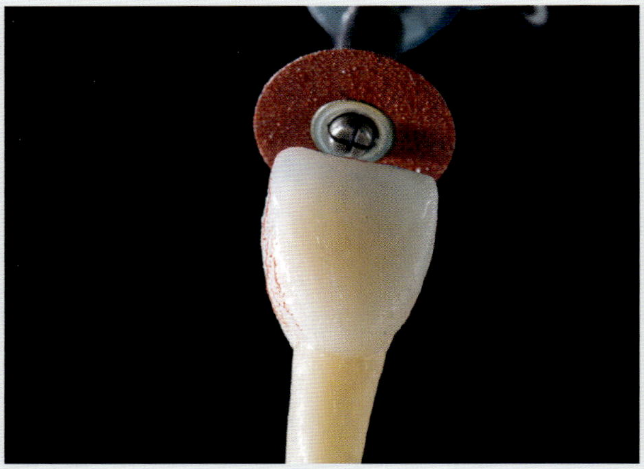

Figure 6 Diamond disc used to regularize the incisal margin.

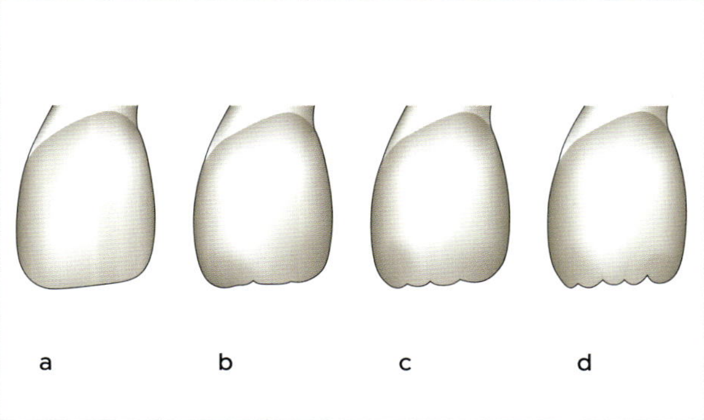

Figure 7 Stylized examples of different degrees of incisal edge irregularity.

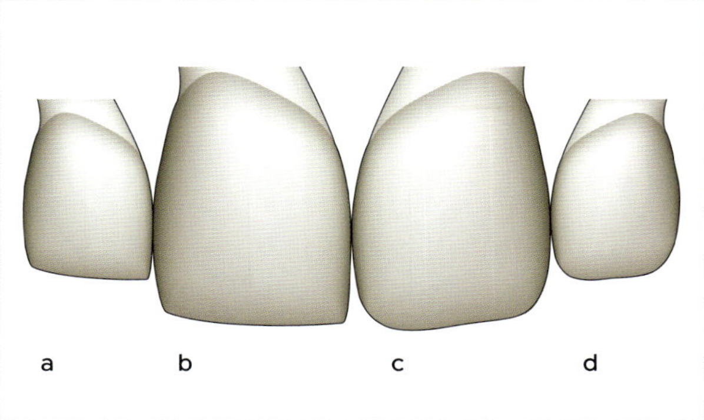

Figure 8 More angular incisal margins (a,b) make the result more "aggressive"; more sinuous margins (c,d) lead to the opposite effect.

Transition lines

As already mentioned, the transition lines play a major role in achieving the final result: they create the light reflections that allow the observer to perceive the three-dimensional morphology of the tooth.

Obviously, in the case of partial restorations, it is essential to ensure that there are no irregularities in the transition lines at the transition point between tooth and composite. If this were the case, even an unobservant observer would immediately notice the error. In the case of complete veneers, as already mentioned, the position of the transition lines can be exploited to create small optical illusions (see 📷 2-4).

In the contouring phase, it is important to highlight the transition lines obtained by modelling, so that it is clear what needs to be done to change them if necessary. The simplest method is to use a lead pencil, passing it sideways along the major convexity of the tooth **(📷 9)**. This will make it possible to draw a line and highlight the shapes.

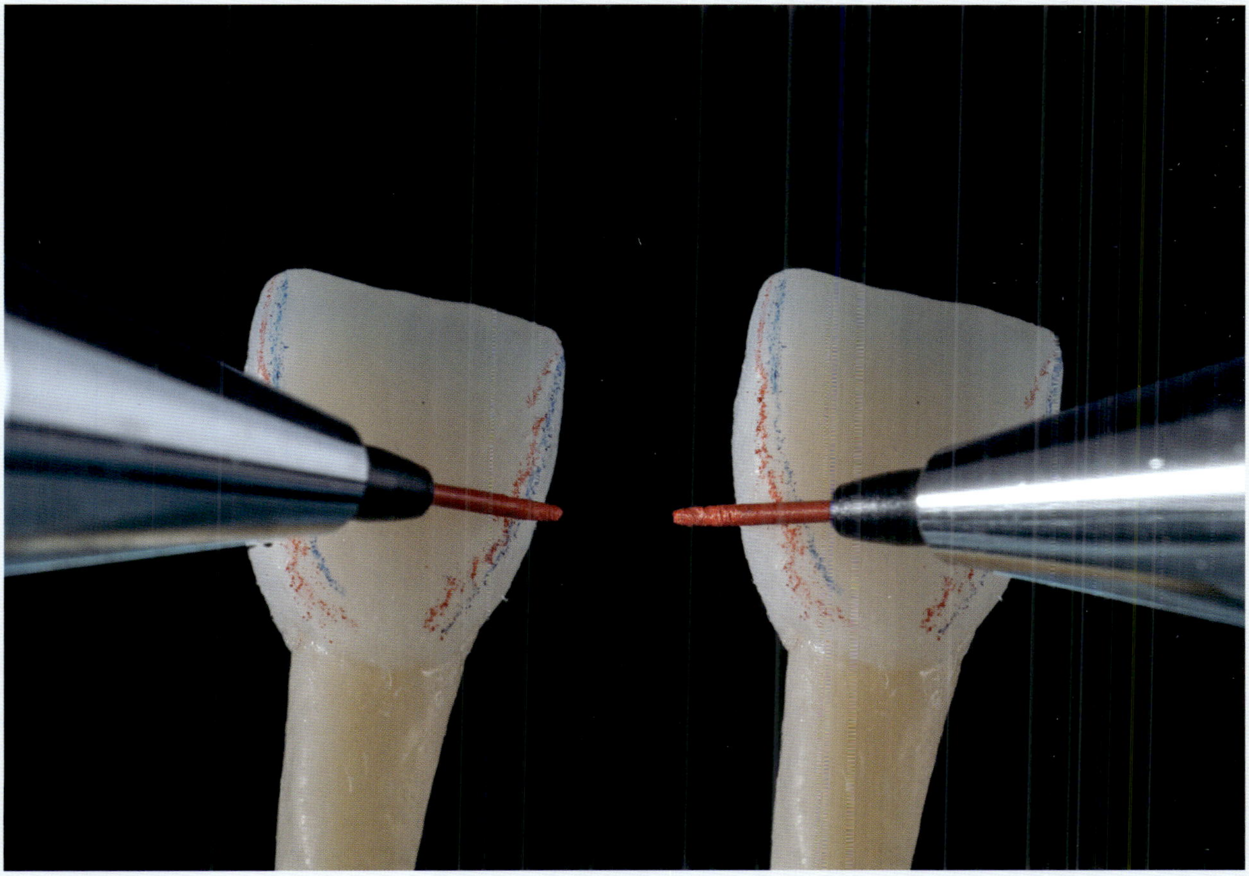

Figure 9 Highlighting the lines executed with modelling. The side of the pencil lead is used.

It may help to mark the position and path of the correct transition line: in this case it is best to use a lead pencil in a different color, drawing with the tip **(📷 10)**. The next picture shows the lines drawn **(📷 11)**.
A coarse- or medium-coarse grit diamond disc can be used to bring the lines from the outside towards the center **(📷 12)**, and a coarse-grained (blue ring perioset) to bring the lines from the center towards the outside **(📷 13)**. In these stages, the coarse-grained cutter on a blue-ring handpiece is preferred to fine-grained cutters on a high-speed handpiece. The greater aggressiveness of the diamond allows the composite to be worked on at low speeds, with great control over the process. In contrast, more delicate cutters require more rotations per minute, making it more difficult to control material removal. Another advantage is the resulting surface roughness, which is useful when

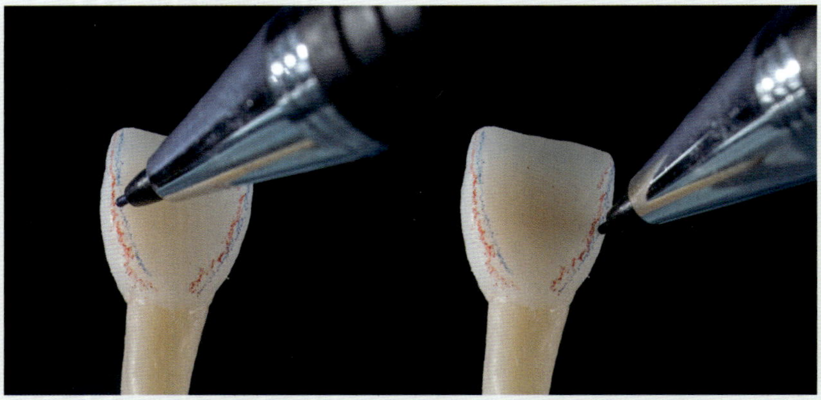

Figure 10 Drawing of the ideal lines to be obtained with contouring. The tip of the pencil lead is used.

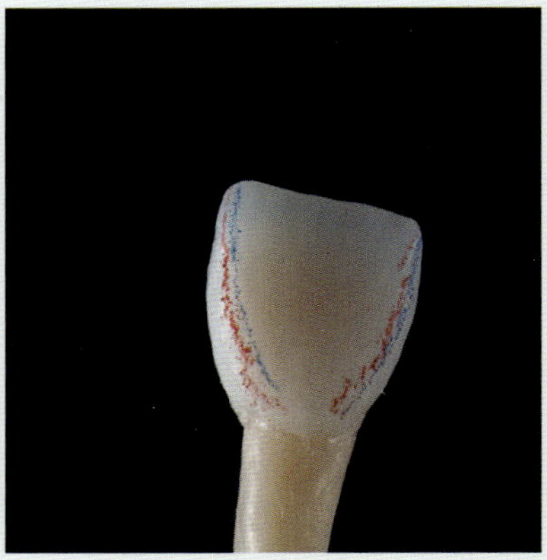

Figure 11 The lines drawn.

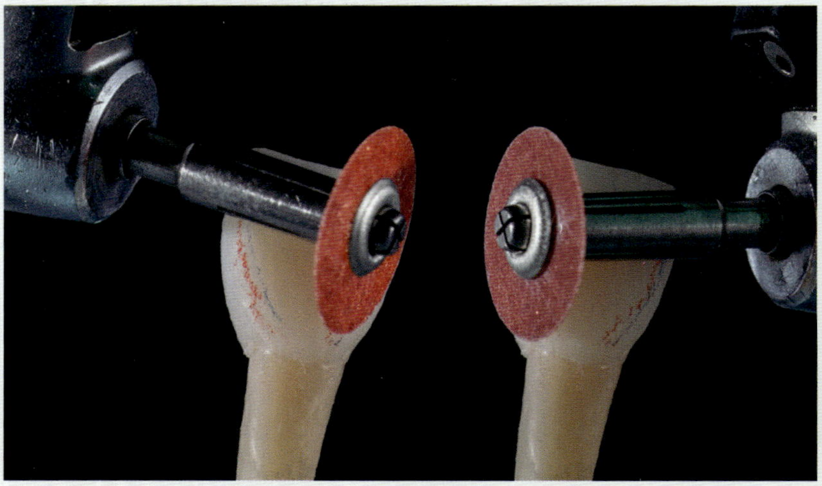

Figure 12 Correction using the pad.

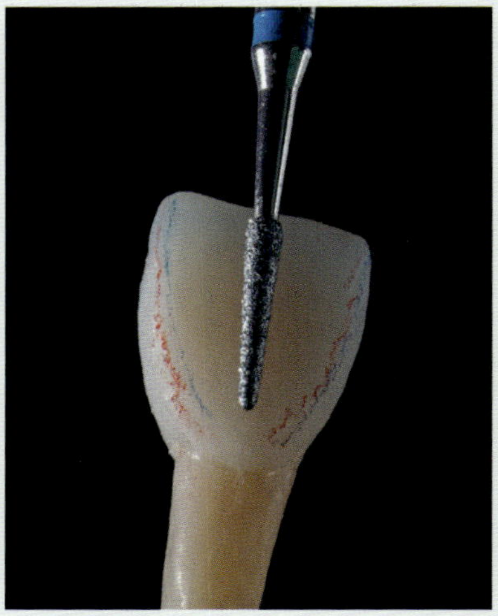

Figure 13 Correction using a milling cutter coarse-grained (blue ring perioset).

creating the surface texture. After the correction (14a), it is good practice to mark the transition lines again with the pencil lead (14b) to assess the need for further work.

Inclination of the vestibular surface

It is also very important to consider the inclination of the buccal surface, according to the planes of the cervical, middle and incisal third. It can be helpful, especially to make the surfaces homogeneous between one tooth and another, to mark the limits between the planes obtained by modelling with a pencil lead, and the ideal limits with a pencil lead of another color (15). A blue ring perioset bur is very useful to redefine the planes, following the indications of the lines (16).

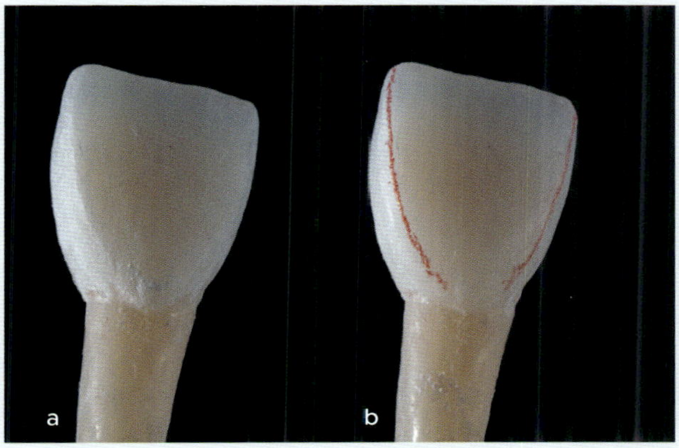

Figure 14 Checking the transition lines after contouring passes.

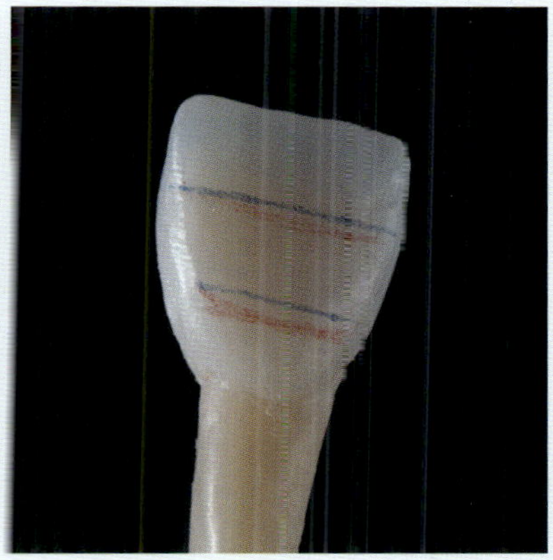

Figure 15 The obtained planes are marked in red, the ideal planes in blue.

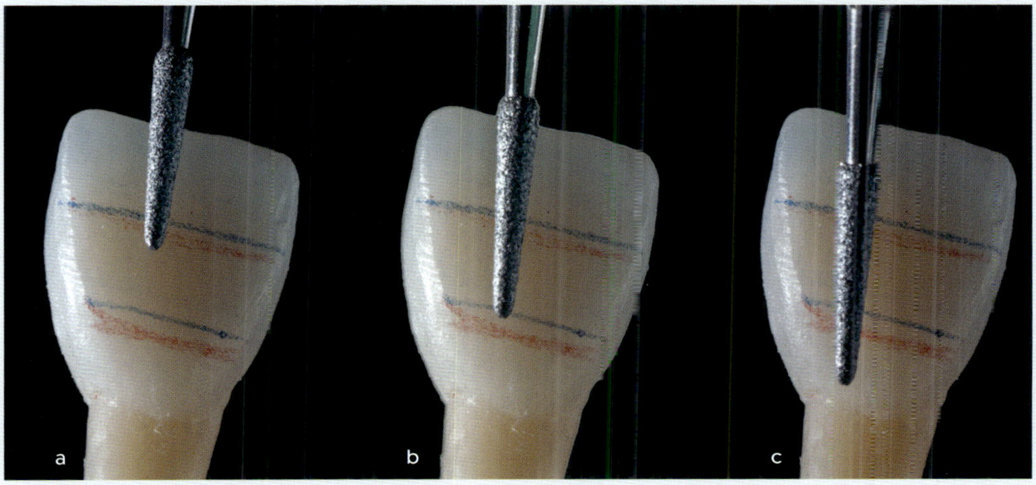

Figure 16 The bur follows the three planes: incisal (a), middle (b) and cervical (c).

FINISHING

In this phase, the surface finishing of the restoration is considered, defining the secondary and tertiary anatomy of the tooth.

Secondary anatomy

We can find different degrees of definition of secondary anatomy in nature, the so-called surface macrotexture. These are vertical depressions due to the growth lobes. They can be more or less intense and generally tend to fade with time and tissue wear. In order to define the secondary anatomy, we can help ourselves once again by tracing the limits of the lobes and depressions with a pencil (📷 17).

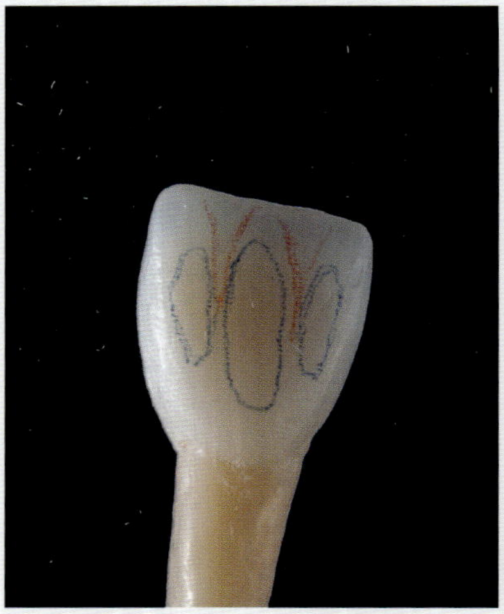

Figure 17 The lobes are marked in blue and the depressions in red.

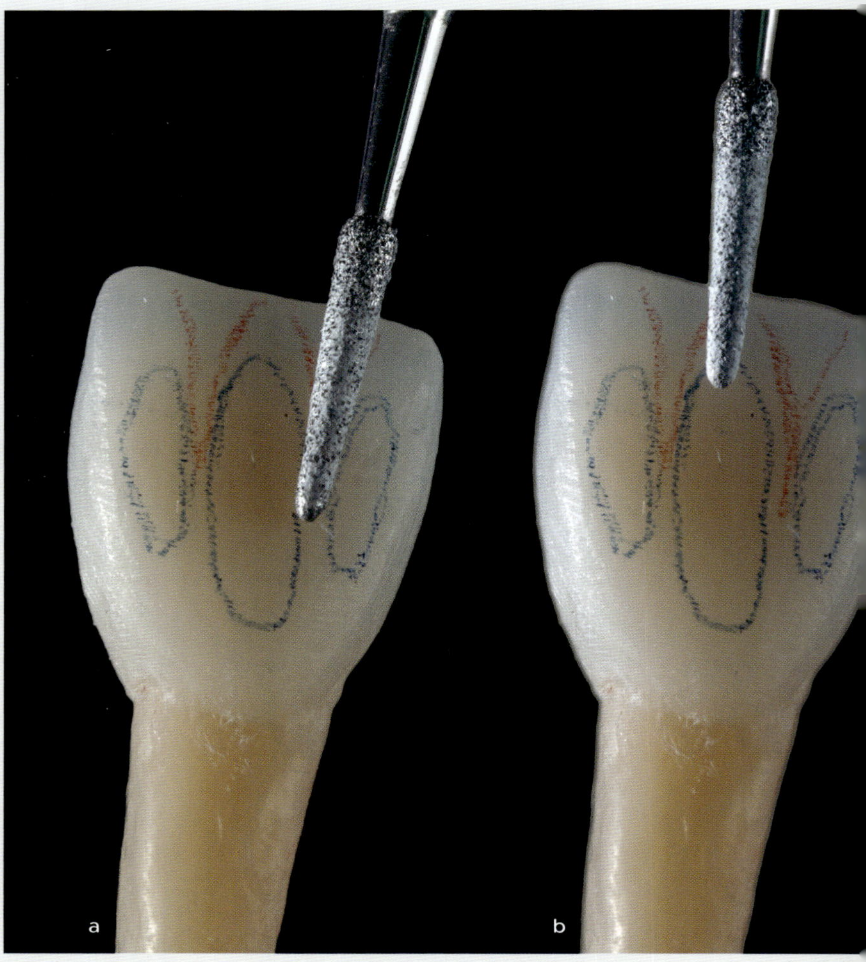

Also, at this stage it is important to try to have as much control as possible over the abrasive instruments, using coarse-grained diamond burs on a blue handpiece. In particular, both the perioset bur and a pellet allow the depressions to be traced very delicately, without the risk of removing too much material by mistake **(18)**.

Tertiary anatomy

Horizontal development furrows create more or less intense striations on the surface, which can be almost straight, curved or wavy. These are called perikymata and are responsible for the surface microtexture. Although they appear to be a minimal detail, they are very important for aesthetic purposes, as they affect the way light is reflected. A partial restoration that is correct in terms of color and primary and secondary anatomy, but does not imitate the microtexture of the natural tooth, cannot be said to be perfectly integrated.

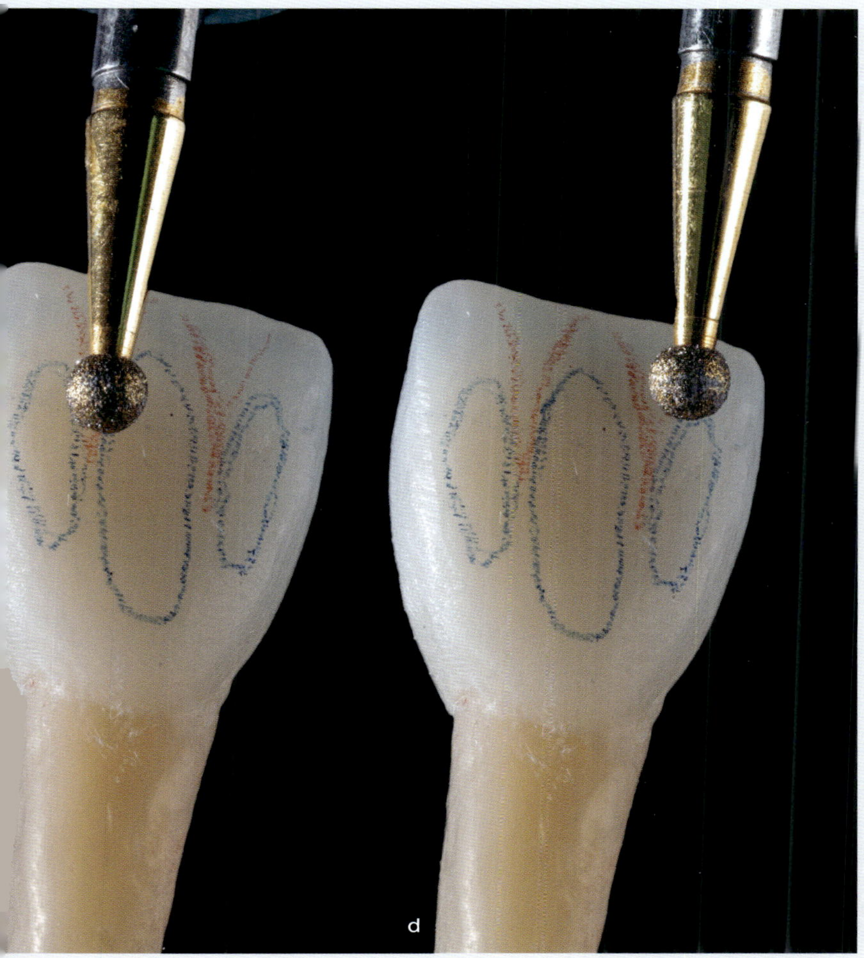

Figure 18 The spear bur (a,b) and the ball (c,d) used to define the secondary anatomy.

Clinical case

The patient had an incongruous restoration on tooth 2.1 (19a), which was removed to make a new composite restoration (19b). Contouring was immediately performed, while it was decided to carry out only a cursory polishing, pending the post-rehydration color check (19c). As can be seen, the lack of surface texture makes it easy to identify the restoration, which has not integrated at all. At the next appointment, once the color correctness has been verified, the finishing steps with the blue ring perioset bur and polishing are carried out. Striae imitating the tertiary anatomy of the natural tooth allow a better integration of the restoration (19d).

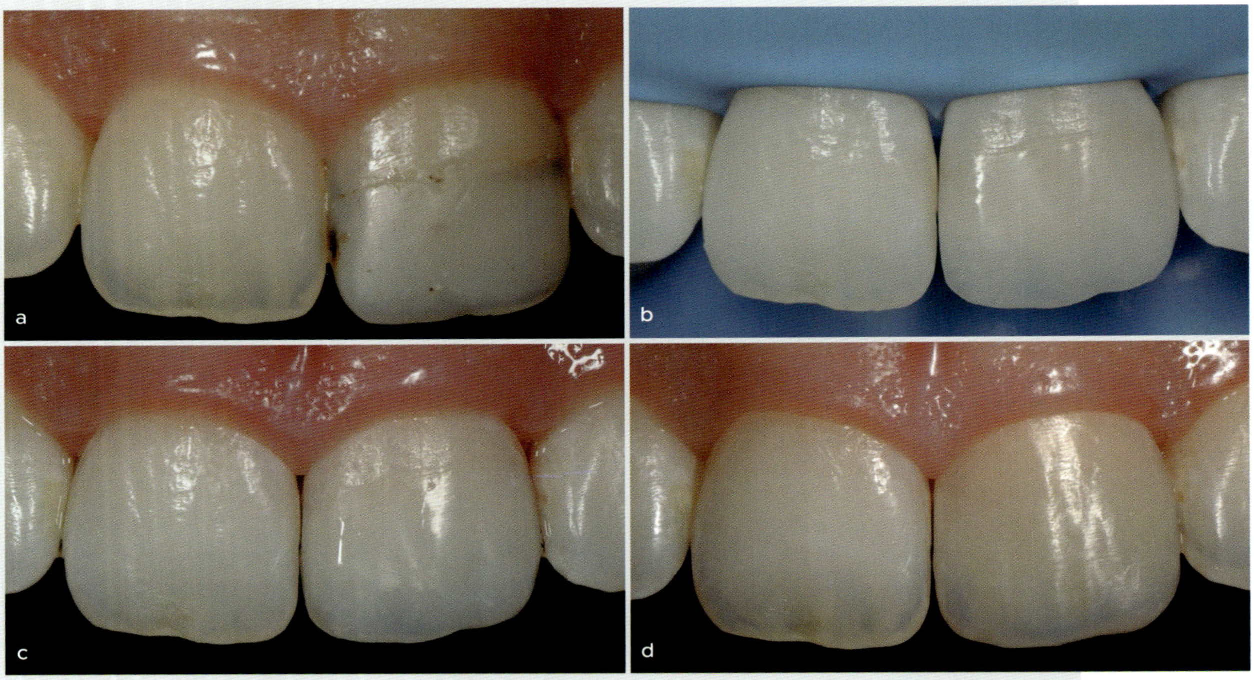

Figure 19 Clinical case highlighting the importance of microtexture. Initial case (a), finished layering (b), polishing without microtexture (c), control photo after creating the texture (d).

In the case of partial restorations one must, of course, try to replicate the tertiary anatomy of the tooth; in the case of complete veneers the clinician has more freedom of action and can simplify the procedure considerably.
In cases where the striae are large and sinuous, the path can be traced with the pencil lead and then acted upon with the tip of the blue ring perioset bur (20).
If the striae are small and sharp, we can use the same coarse-grained bur but working it with the body (21b). The large diamond will create the tertiary anatomy very easily. The movement will be in a horizontal direction, with a straight or curved path depending on the course of the striae we want to reproduce: for this it may be useful to trace the path with the pencil lead (21a).

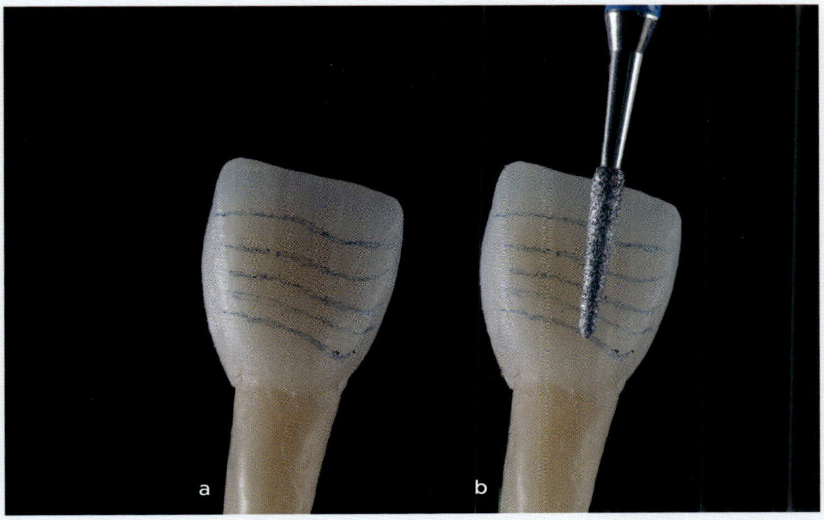

Figure 20 The lines drawn for wide grooves (a) are traced with the blue ring perioset drill bit (b).

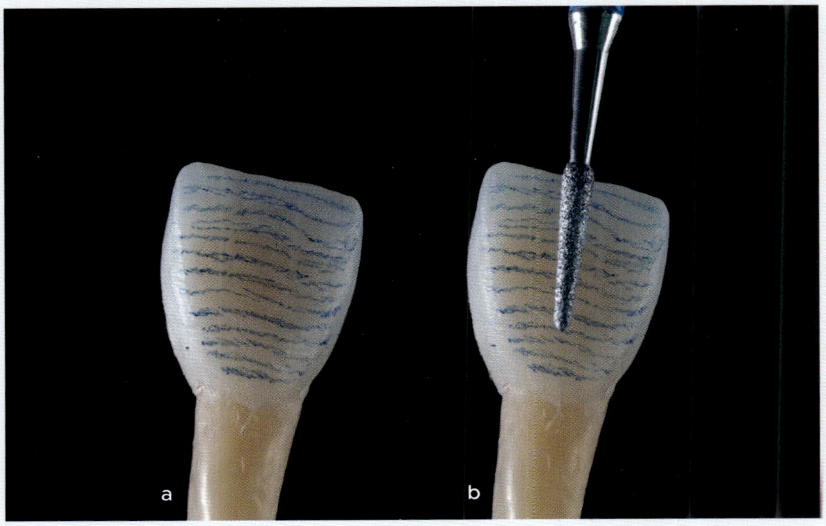

Figure 21 The lines drawn for fine grooves are traced with the drill bit (a), so that a direction can be followed with the horizontal movement of the blue ring perioset cutter, which works with the body (b).

POLISHING

The characteristics of the fillers in modern composites often make polishing easy. In many cases it is sufficient to use medium-abrasiveness silicone tips **(📷 22a)** or discs **(📷 22b)** and, by calibrating the pressure and speed of rotation, adjust the intensity of the action. Care must always be taken not to overheat the tooth, as the low abrasive tool creates a lot of friction and, consequently, heat.

Brilliant polishing

The final and equally delicate step is polishing. This procedure will not only result in a shinier and brighter surface, but also better preservation over time, with less pigment retention. StyleItaliano has developed a polishing kit called Lucida, consisting of a very fine-grained (sub-micron) water-soluble paste called Lucida Paste **(📷 23a)**, and a star-shaped felt, called Lucida Star **(📷 23b)**. The special shape of the felt allows a fully automatic intermittent action and the possibility of reaching areas that are difficult to polish with traditional devices. The low cost allows them to be used as disposables, circumventing the problem of the difficult cleaning of normal felts, which poorly withstand the high temperatures of autoclaves.
The following pictures **(📷 24-27)** show the results obtained.

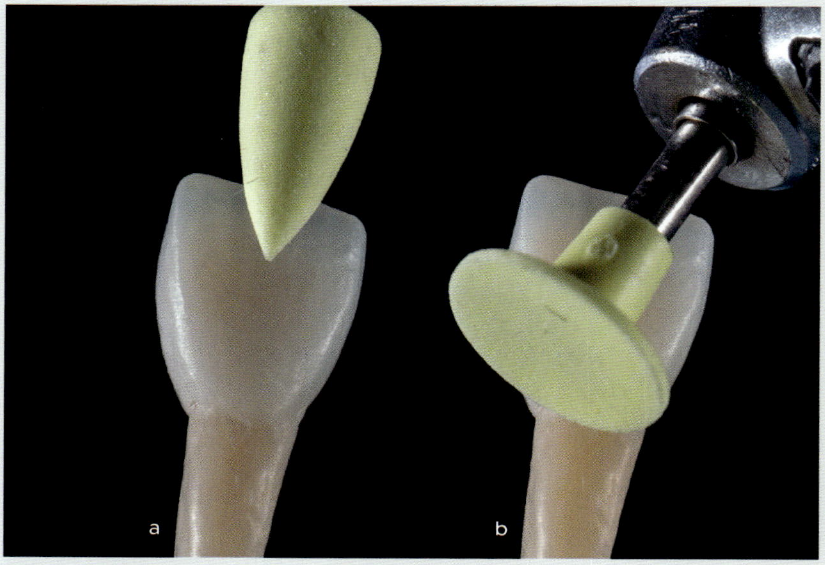

Figure 22 Tips (a) or discs (b) in silicone can be used for the first polishing step.

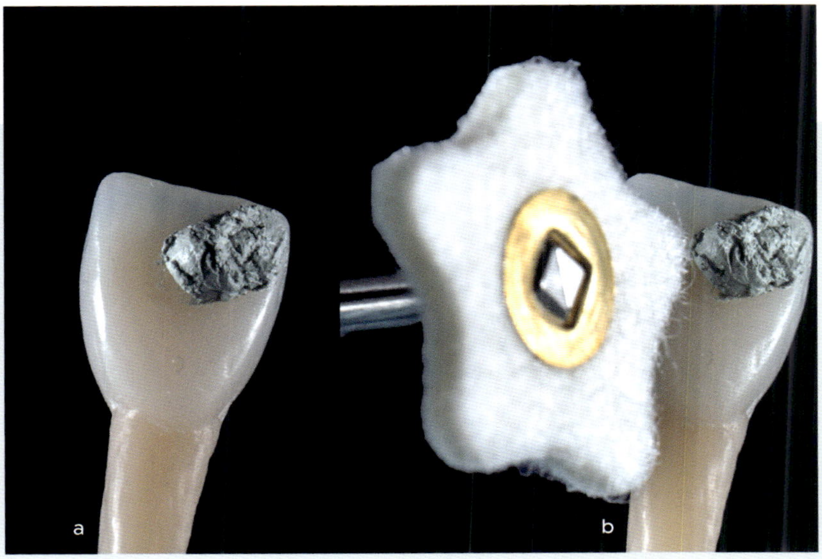

Figure 23 Lucida Paste applied in a small amount on the surface to be treated (a), and Lucida Star in place to begin the procedure (b).

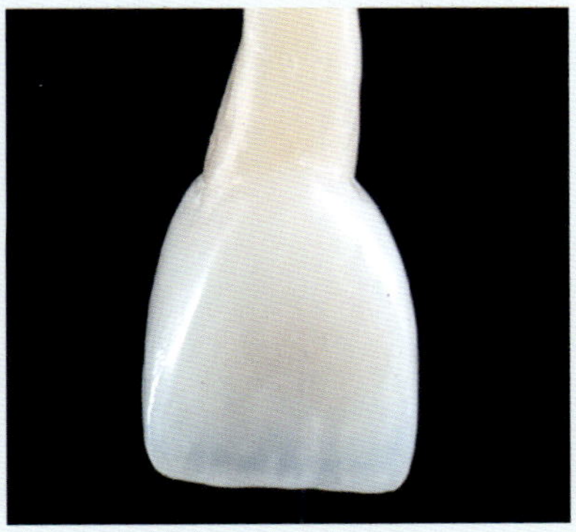

Figure 24 Front view of the tooth.

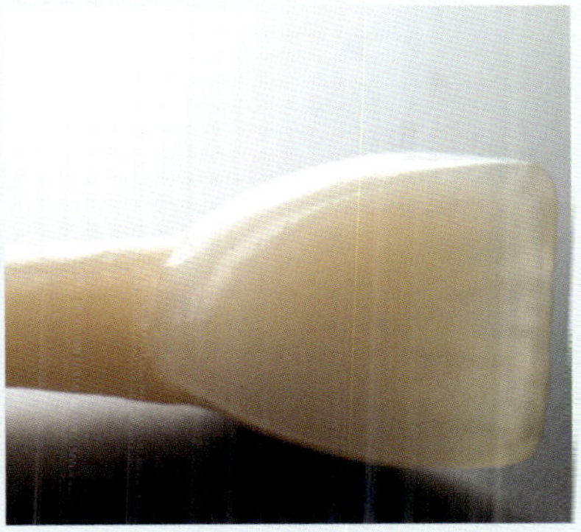

Figure 25 The tooth with transmitted light.

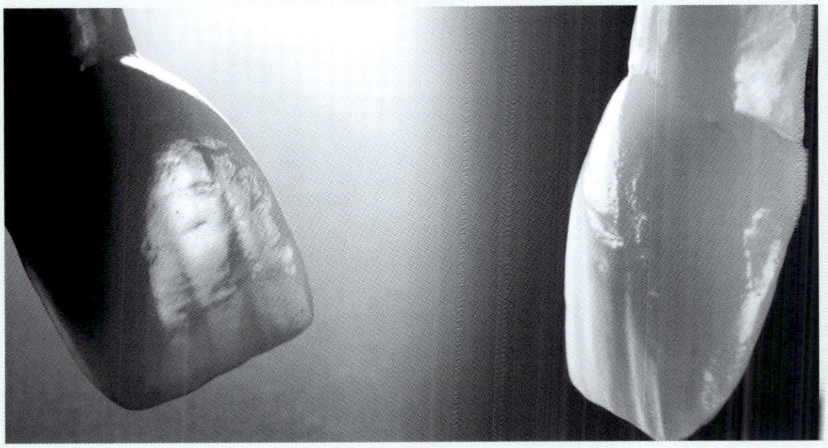

Figure 26 The greyscale image helps to better understand the chiaroscuro, and thus to interpret the surface morphology.

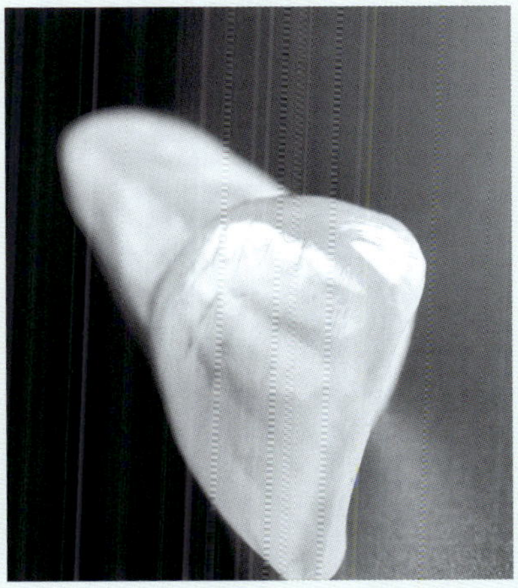

Figure 27 Another useful angle to better understand the texture.

Clinical case 1

The patient presented complaining of an unsightly old composite restoration on tooth 1.1 (28a). It was decided to remove it and replace it with a new direct restoration. After isolating the surgical field with the rubber dam, the old restoration was removed and the preparation polished (28b). Then the adhesive procedures were carried out and the composite was layered until the new restoration was obtained (28c).

The contouring phase begins with the blue perioset bur (28d) to define the transition lines, and the red perioset (28e) to better smooth the surfaces.

To better highlight the three-dimensionality of the surface, a blue articulating paper was rubbed onto the vestibular surface of the tooth (28f). A diamond bur was then used for secondary anatomy (28g) and a silicone polisher for initial polishing (28h). Final polishing was performed with Lucida Paste (28i) and Lucida Star (28j). The final result (28k) was photographed at one-month follow-up (28l).

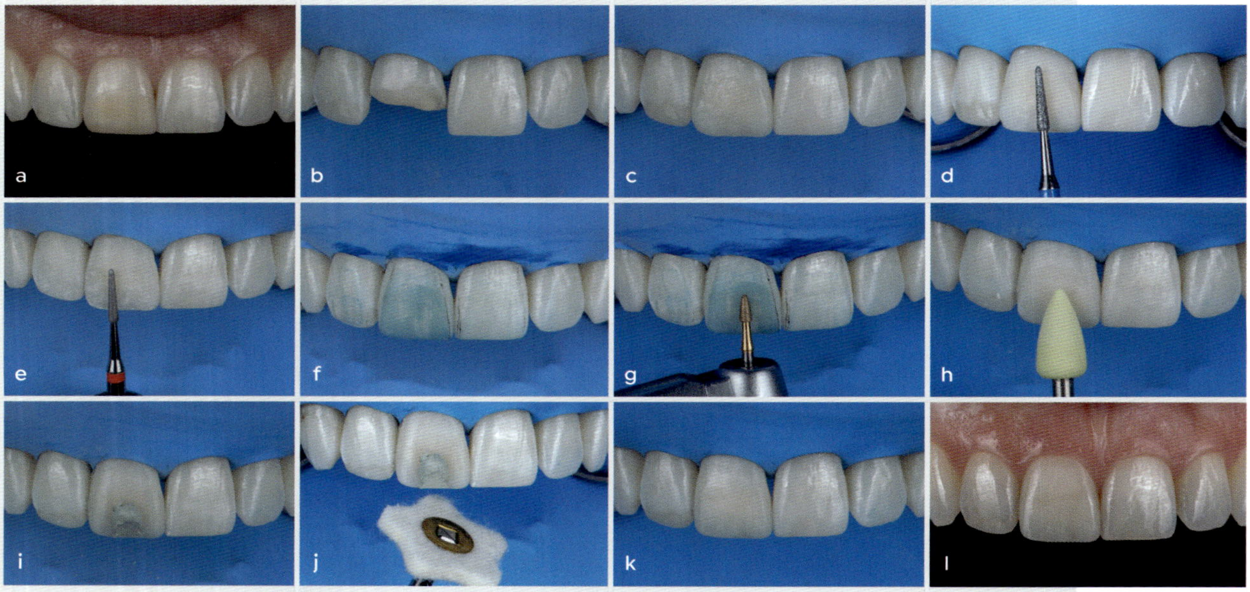

Figure 28 Step-by-step finishing of a Class IV restoration of tooth 1.1. Initial photo (a), restoration removed (b), new restoration (c), blue perioset (d), red perioset (e), surface highlighting with articulating paper (f), secondary anatomy (g), initial polish (h), Lucida Paste (i), Lucida Star (j), polished restoration (k), one-month follow-up (l).

Clinical case 2

The patient was sent to an orthodontist colleague with a request to close the diastemas and improve the shape. As can be seen from the picture (29, 30a), she also has two old composite restorations on the lateral conoids.

Given the patient's young age it is decided to proceed with direct composite restorations. All data were collected and shared with the laboratory to create a wax-up, through which a mock-up can be performed. Once the design was validated, we moved on to the operative phase.

After isolating the field with the rubber dam, we started working on the two central incisors, expanding the isolation with two B4 clamps (30b). The surfaces are sandblasted with aluminum oxide (Aquacare Twin) to be prepared for adhesion (30c). With the help of an instrument that functions as both retractor and matrix (LM Gengiva) the new enamel-cement junctions were created one by one (30d). The restorations were then finished according to the usual procedures (30e) and the contouring, finishing and polishing steps were carried out.

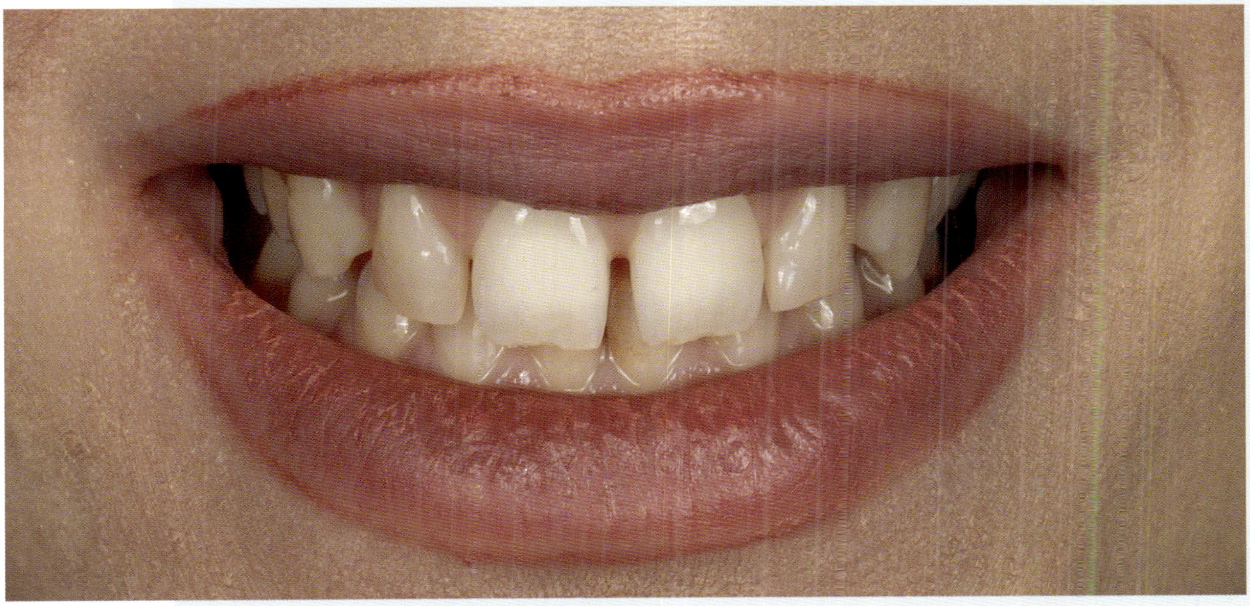

Figure 29 The patient's smile before reconstructions.

At follow-up the restorations are well integrated (📷 30f-h) and the remarkable aesthetic change can be seen by comparing the pre- and post-operative images (📷 31).

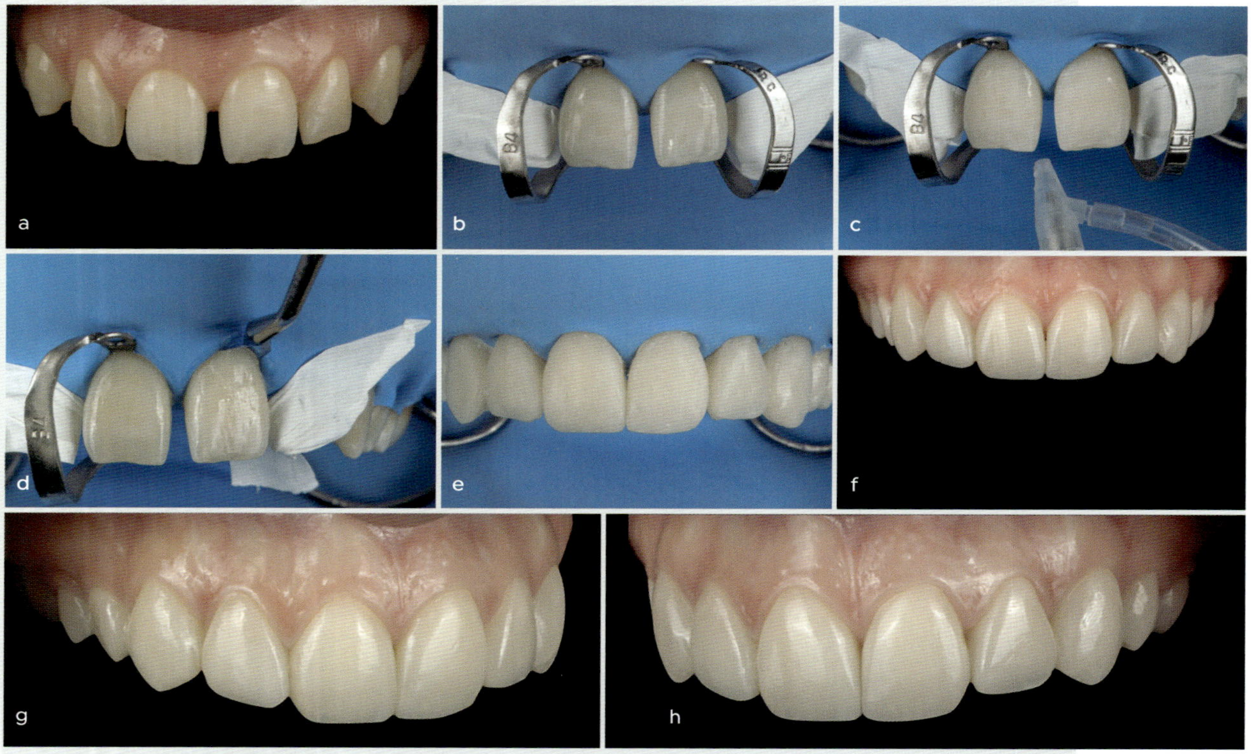

Figure 30 Initial photo (a), isolation (b), treatment surface (c), new CEJs (d), completed restoration (e), follow-up at one month (f-h).

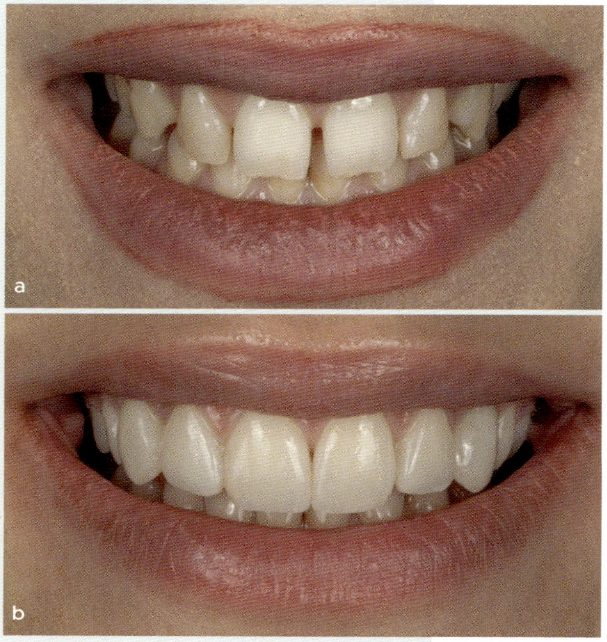

Figure 31 Comparison of before and after restorations.

CONCLUSION

We have seen how the finishing stages of the restoration play a major role in achieving a good result. What might seem to be a marginal part instead needs time, attention, dedicated techniques and tools, especially when we are talking about partial restorations, in which it is mandatory to imitate the characteristics of the restored tooth.

In cases of complete veneering of the whole area, of course, the clinicians can allow themself more freedom in creating macro- and micro-anatomies.

The procedure has a certain degree of complexity, but it is by no means complicated. By knowing the correct protocols, everyone can achieve an excellent result in daily clinical practice.

A great contribution comes from photography. Direct observation (with and without magnification systems) can lead the clinician to a partial reading of the situation. By photographing the various stages, and immediately checking the photo on the camera screen, the clinician can see much more detail, given the absence of stereoscopic vision and the possibility of greatly enlarging the image.

SUGGESTED READINGS

- Devoto W, Saracinelli M, Manauta J. Composite in everyday practice: how to choose the right material and simplify application techniques in the anterior teeth. *Eur J Esthet Dent.* 2010;5(1):102-124.
- Manauta J, Salat A. *Layers. An atlas of composite resin stratification.* Quintessence Publishing, 2012.
- Manauta J, Salat A, Devoto W, Putignano A. *Layers 2. Direct composites: the Styleitaliano clinical secrets.* Quintessence Publishing 2023.
- Rufenacht C-R. *Principles of Esthetic Integration.* Quintessence Publishing, 2000.

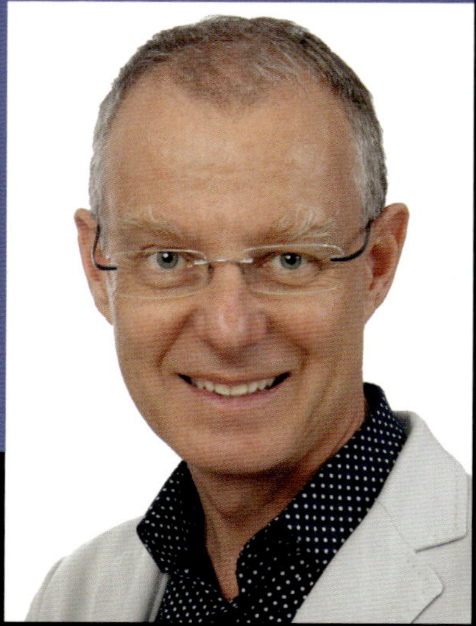

MONALDO SARACINELLI

Italy

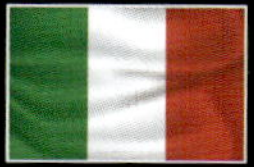

Monaldo Saracinelli was born in 1958. He was Lecturer on the Master's Degree in Endodontics and Restorative Dentistry at the University of Siena; Lecturer at the Faculté d'Odontologie Aix Marseille Université (France); Lecturer at the Dentistry Student Conference, Pharos University in Alexandria (Egypt); Lecturer at the Diplôme d'Odontologie Esthétique, Université de Montpellier (France); Visiting Professor at the University of Padua in the Postgraduate Master's Course in Paediatric Dentistry and Early Orthodontic Treatments. He has been an active member of the AIC (Italian Academy of Conservative Dentistry), the IAED (Italian Academy of Esthetic Dentistry) and the StyleItaliano group since its foundation.

Author and co-author of several publications in international scientific journals, he is a speaker at national and international courses and congresses. He carries out his clinical practice

SHAPE ANOMALIES. CONSERVATIVE APPROACH WITH DIRECT TECHNIQUE

Aesthetic problems of the anterior sector caused by abnormalities in shape and size, often due to congenital changes during the dental developmental stage, can result in significant smile problems, especially in young female patients, interfering with their social relationships. The best approach, based on both age and future changes due to growth, is undoubtedly a solution that is non-invasive, reversible and respectful of dental tissues, taking advantage of adhesive techniques and the aesthetic resolution possibilities offered by modern composite materials.
The direct reconstructive approach also offers the possibility of future re-interventions for maintenance, correction and repair, with the undoubted advantage of postponing more expensive and invasive prosthetic techniques over time. On the other hand, many colleagues complain that the layering techniques are complex and the choice of color arduous; paradoxically, they report greater difficulty with the introduction on the market of sophisticated materials aimed at optimizing the final result in the medium and long term.
This contribution discusses these issues and provides suggestions for achieving a satisfactory result from an aesthetic and clinical point of view, but above all predictable. This leads to undeniable advantages in terms of quality of work and economy for both us and our patients.

DISCUSSION AND CLINICAL CASE

The 16-year-old female patient, dissatisfied with her smile, comes to the office for prosthetic treatment aimed at shape transformation of both upper lateral incisors, which are different from each other and smaller than normal in size **(📷 1)**, as well as affected by small diastemas with the central incisors and canines **(📷 2)**.

The treatment plan, after a thorough oral hygiene session and motivational reinforcement of the patient, continues with precision silicone polyvinylsiloxane impressions and occlusal

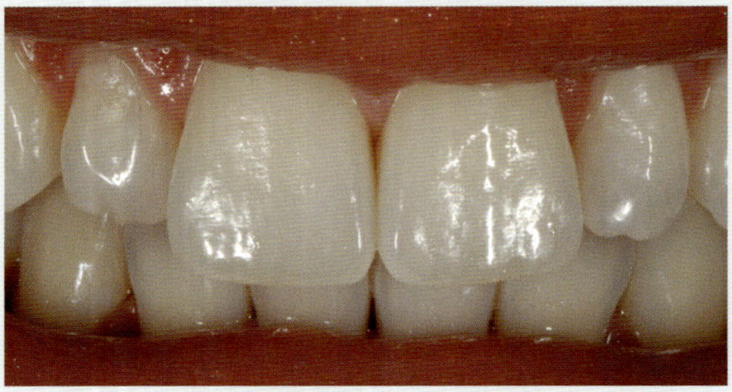

Figure 1 Note the upper lateral incisors, which are different from each other and smaller than normal in size.

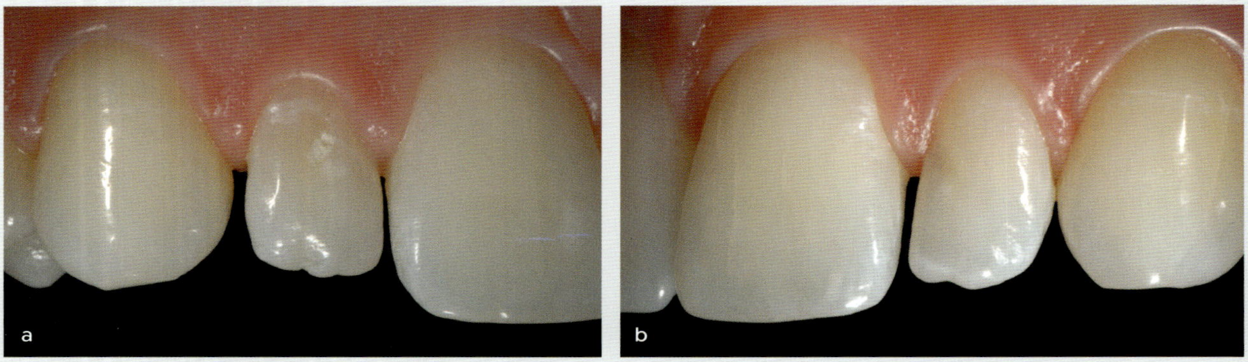

Figure 2 Diastemas with the central incisors and canines.

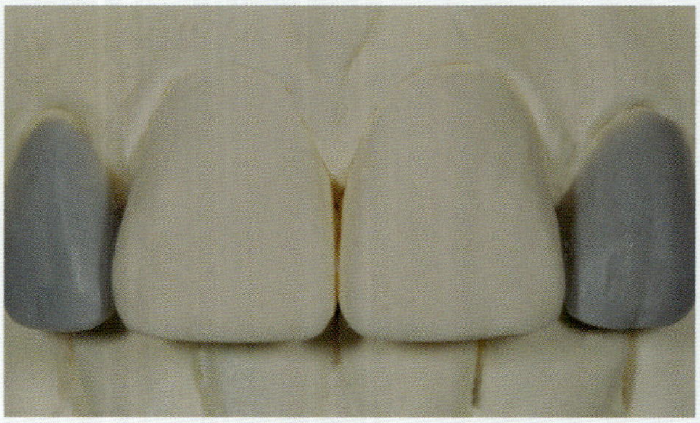

Figure 3 Diagnostic wax-up.

contact registration waxes to assess shape changes of teeth 1.2 and 2.2. Close attention is also paid to the canine disclusion function so that it protects the incisal margins from fracture subsequent to the lengthening of the incisal margin itself. Based on the indications provided, the laboratory technician prepares a diagnostic wax-up (📷 3).

On the plaster model of the diagnostic wax-up, several rigid silicone laboratory templates are made, which are indispensable guides for determining the palatal wall, checking the thickness and layering of the composite masses, and the final shape of the restorations (📷 4).

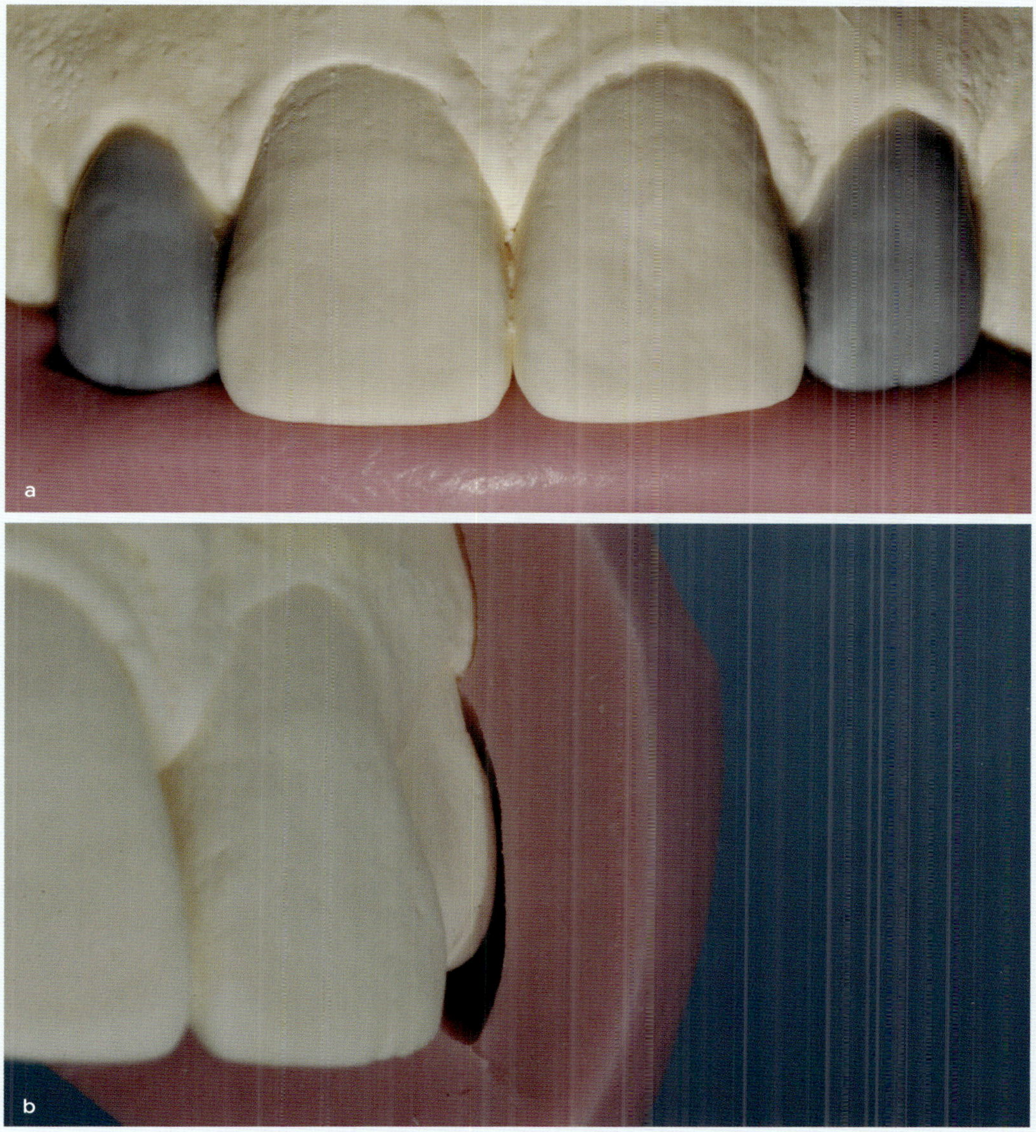

Figure 4 Fabrication of silicone templates on plaster model.

The field isolation with the rubber dam is then made and the template is tested (📷 5, 6). Subsequently, palatal and interproximal boxing is performed to modify the shape in length and to close the diastemas with high-value, low-translucency composite enamel (📷 7).

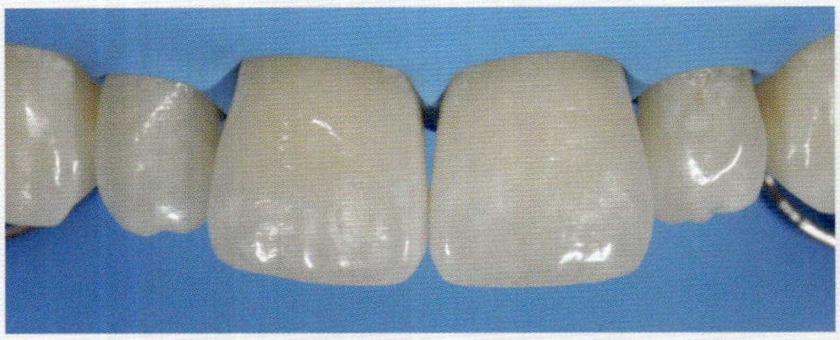

Figure 5 Isolation of the surgical field with rubber dam of medium thickness (Nic Tone).

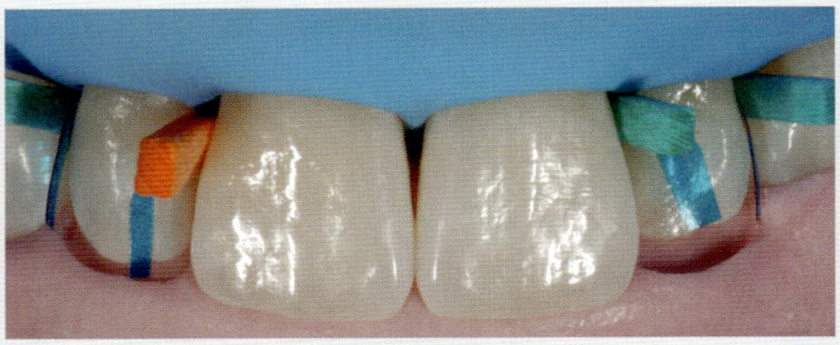

Figure 6 Testing of rigid silicone template with inserted acetate sectional matrices (Hawe Neos).

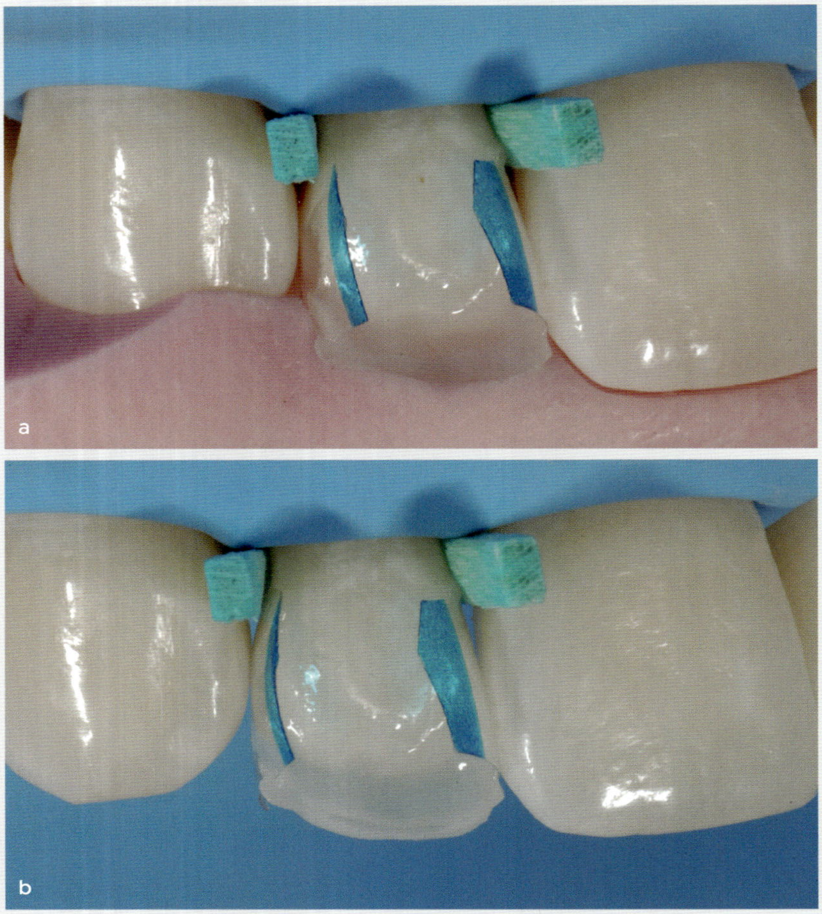

Figure 7 Palatal and interproximal boxing of 1.2.

After contour modification (8), taking advantage of the elasticity of the interproximal matrices that allowed the diastemas to be closed and the emergence profiles of 1.2 and 2.2 (9) – also avoiding cervical overcontours of material – the layering continues with the use of an A1-colored composite dentin mass in the middle and cervical thirds and a high-value enamel in the incisal third to close the restorations (10-14).

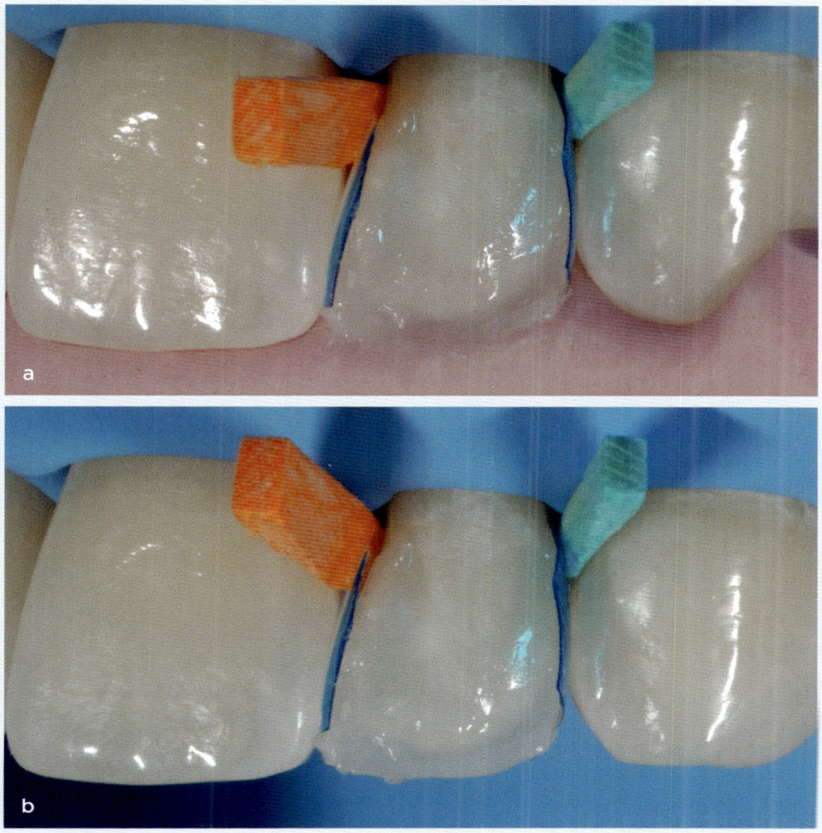

Figure 8 Images of contour shape change after removal of palatal silicone template tooth 2.2.

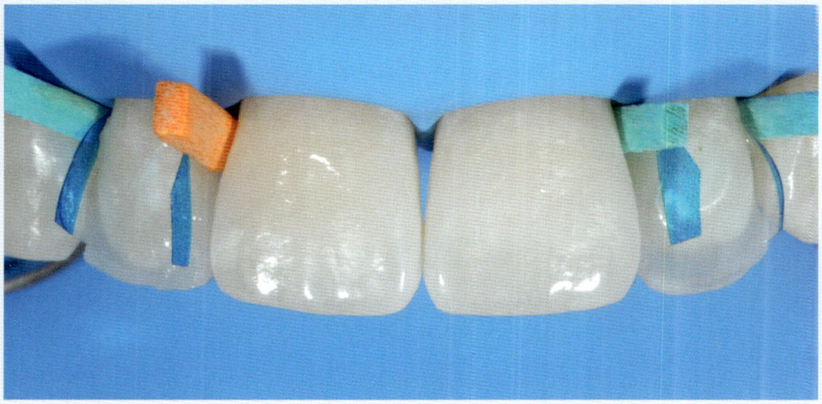

Figure 9 Change in shape and contour of the two teeth.

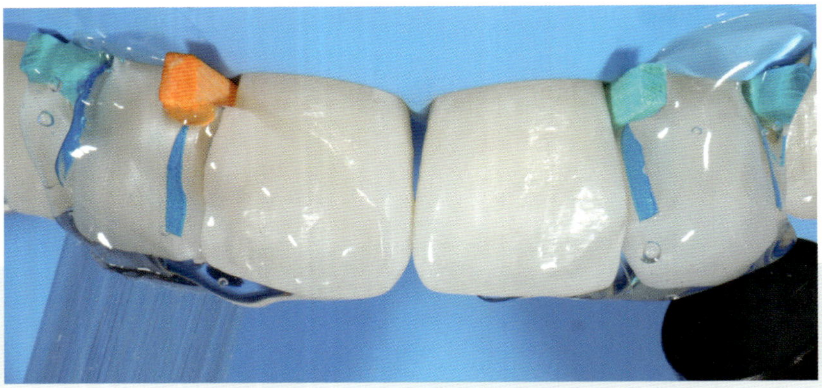

Figure 10 Further cycle polymerization of 60 sec under ultrasonic gel for inhibition of the layer of surface oxygen.

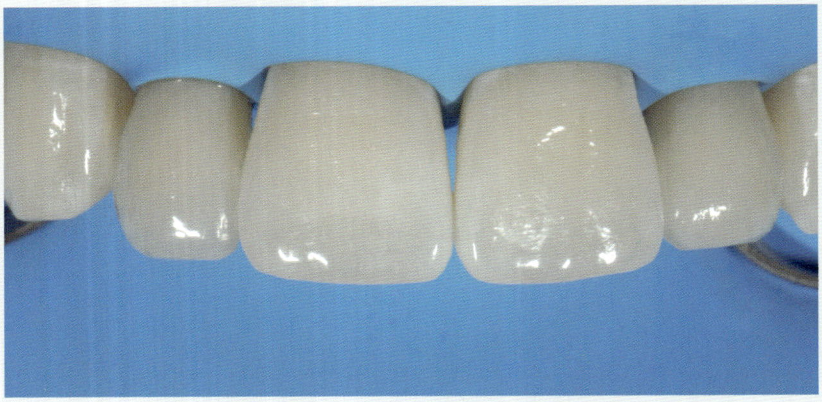

Figure 11 Image of completed restorations, still under dam, after the finishing steps performed with medium- and fine-grain diamond discs and strips on blue low-speed handpiece only in the interproximal corners, of flame diamond burs on red handpiece multiplier of speed on the buccal surface to recreate the surface macro- and microgeography, and of diamond paste polishing with natural bristle brushes and low-speed felts on low-speed blue handpiece.

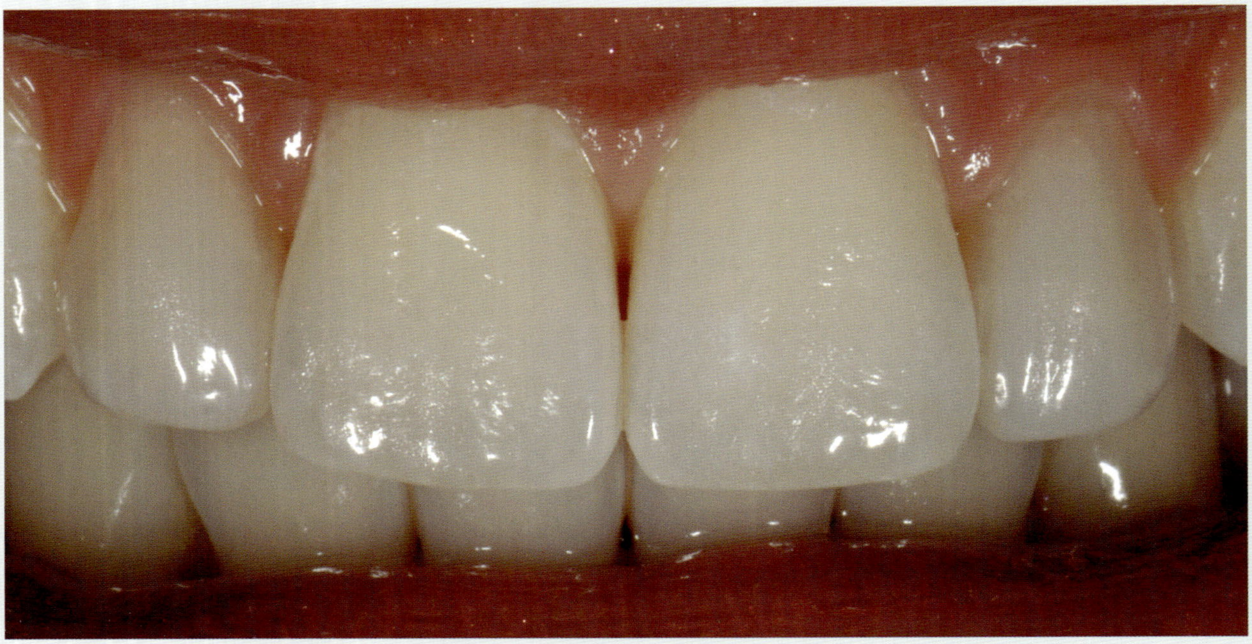

Figure 12 Completed restorations rehydrated two weeks apart. Excellent color and shape integration can be seen.

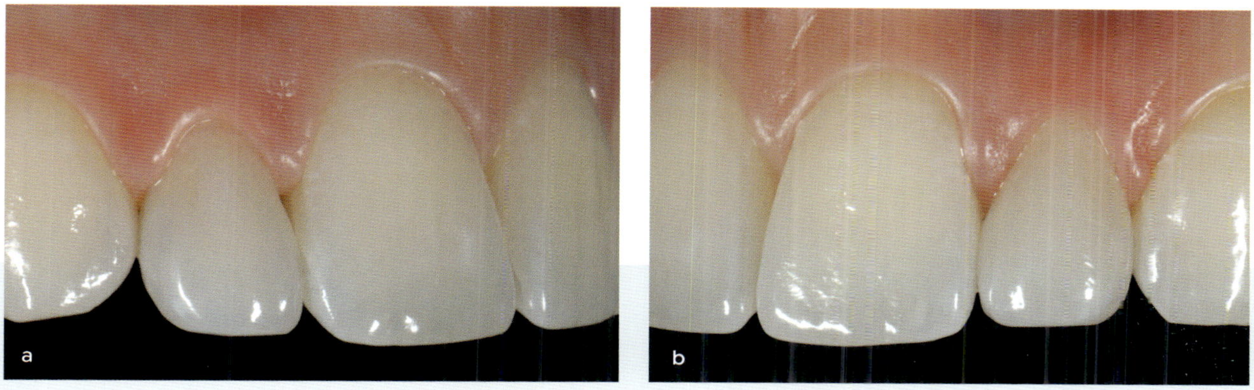

Figure 13 Detail 1.2 and 2.2.

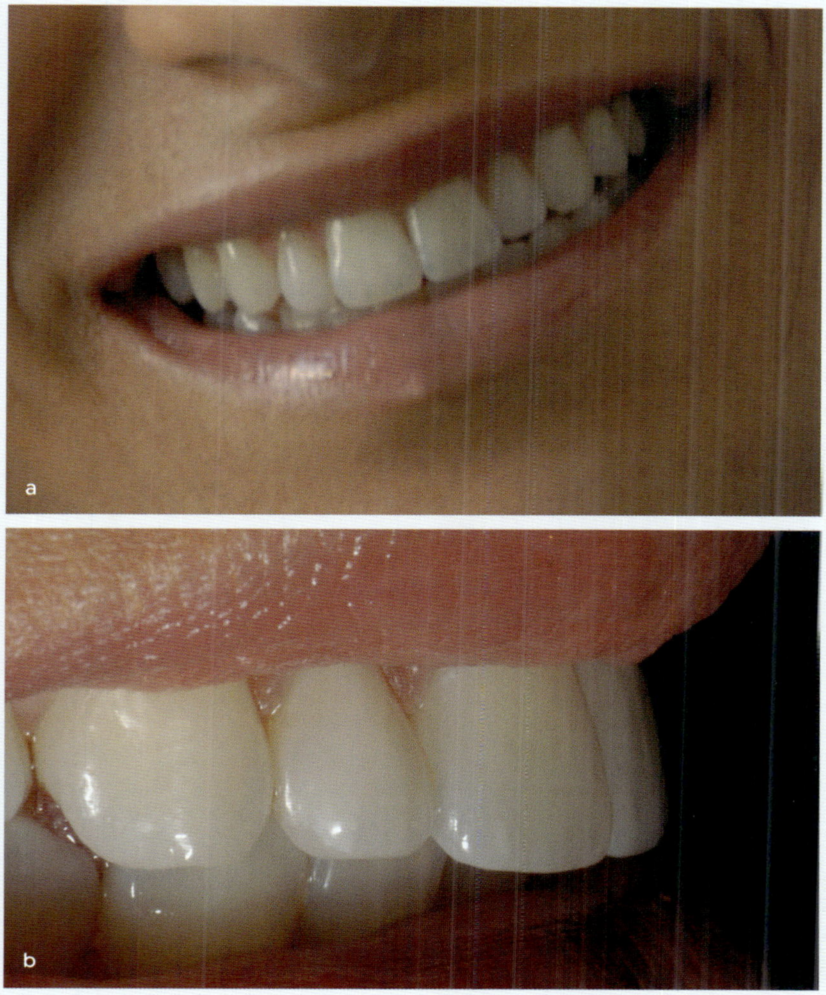

Figure 14 The young patient's new smile.

Follow-ups at 4, 7, 12 and 15 years (📷 15-23) show the perfect fit of the restorations.

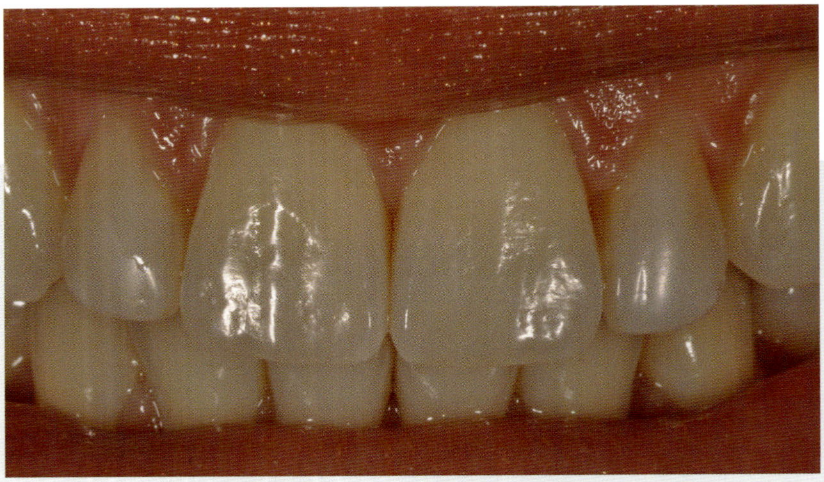

Figure 15 Follow-up at 4 years: superficial opacification with shape retention of the restorations is observed.

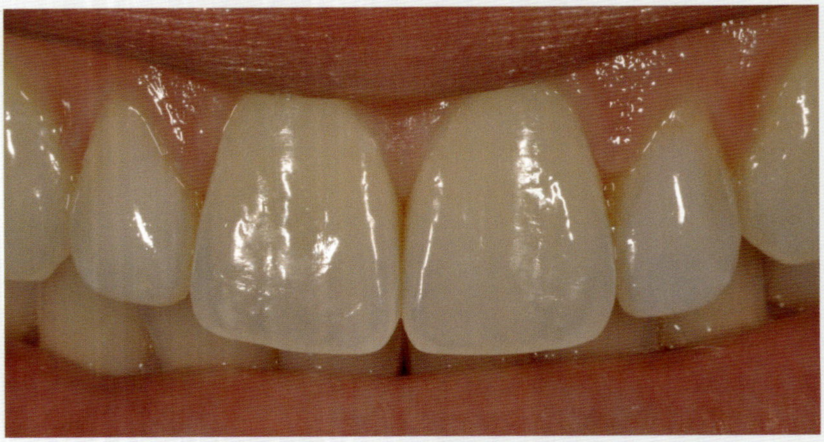

Figure 16 Image at a distance of 4 years after re-polishing with diamond paste.

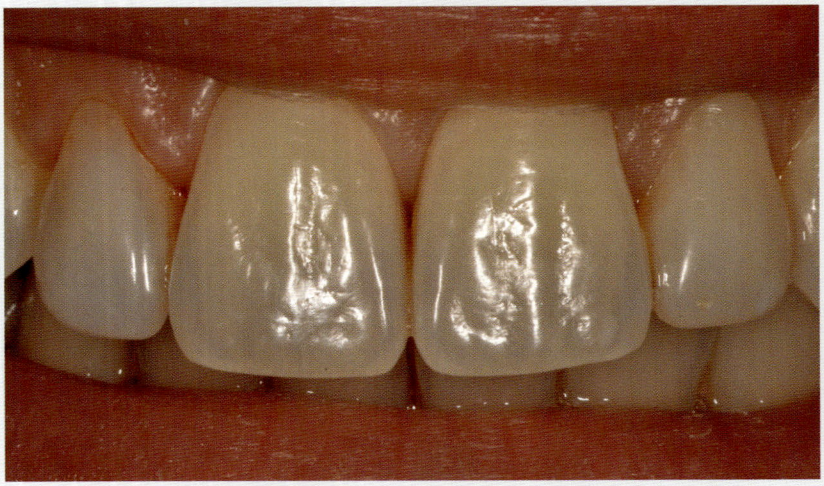

Figure 17 Follow-up at 7 years without further polishing phase.

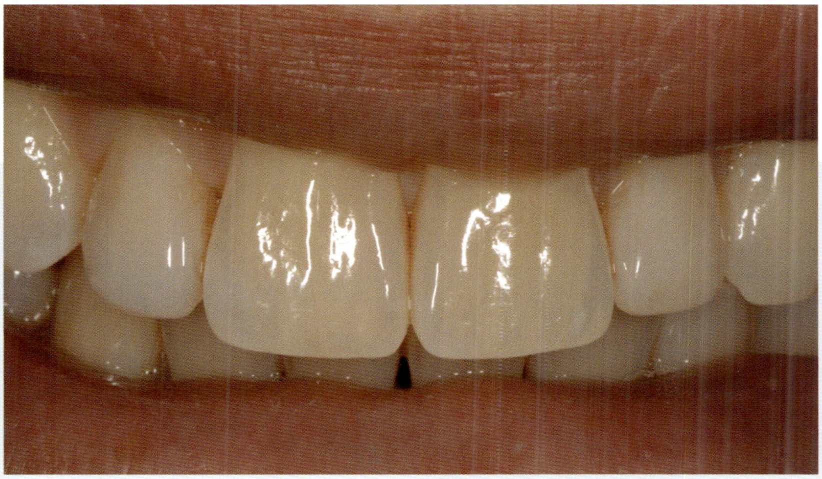

Figure 18 Follow-up at 12 years after re-polishing with diamond paste.

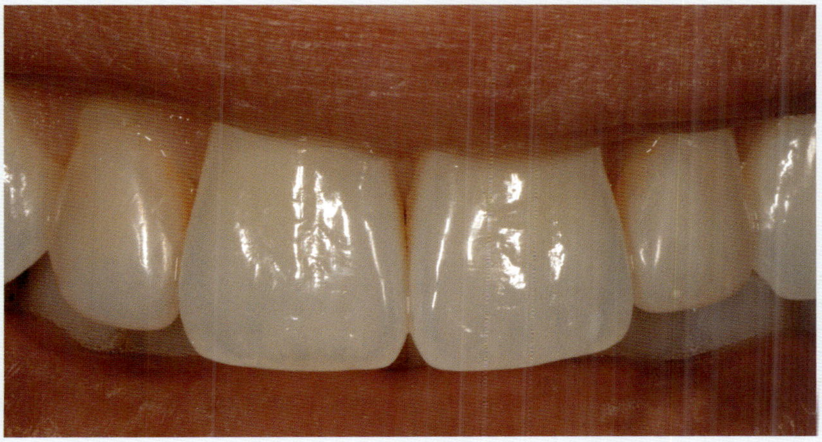

Figure 19 Follow-up at 15 years before of further polishing.

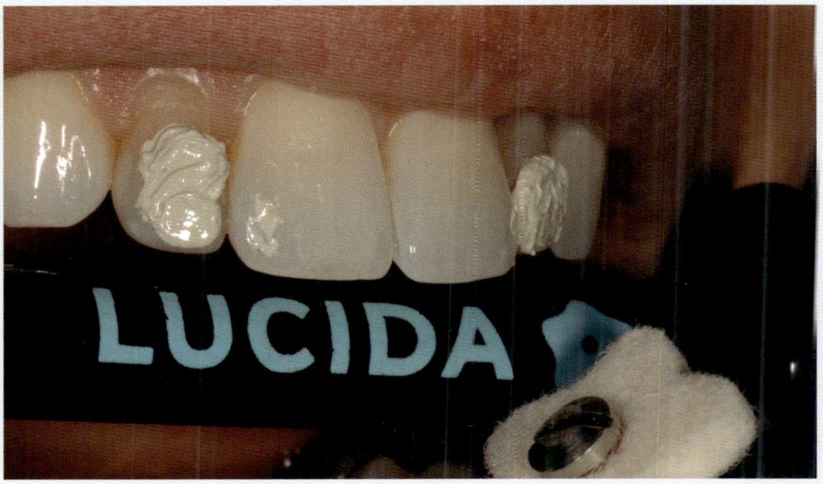

Figure 20 Diamond paste from polishing.

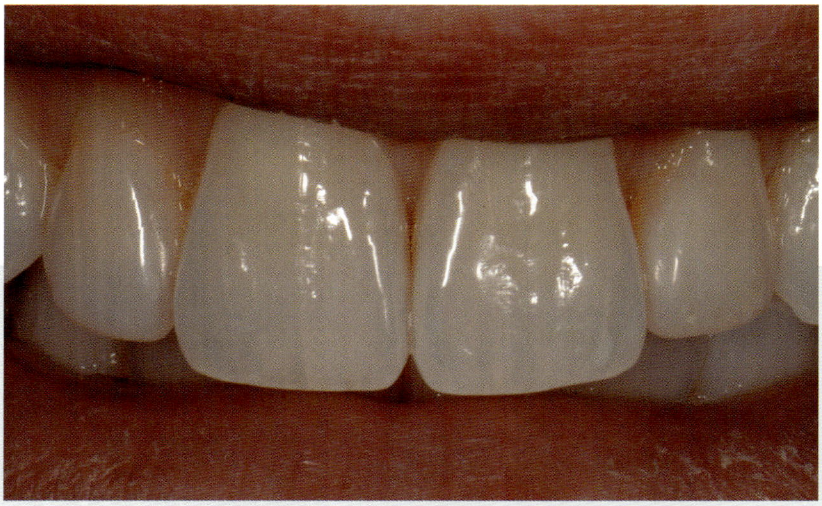

Figure 21 Image at a distance of 15 years after re-polishing with diamond paste.

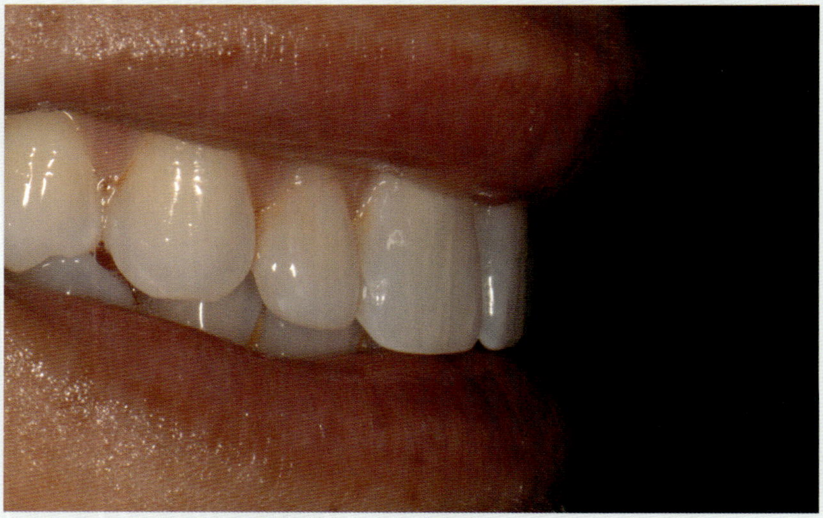

Figure 22 The patient's smile still fully satisfied with the result 15 years later.

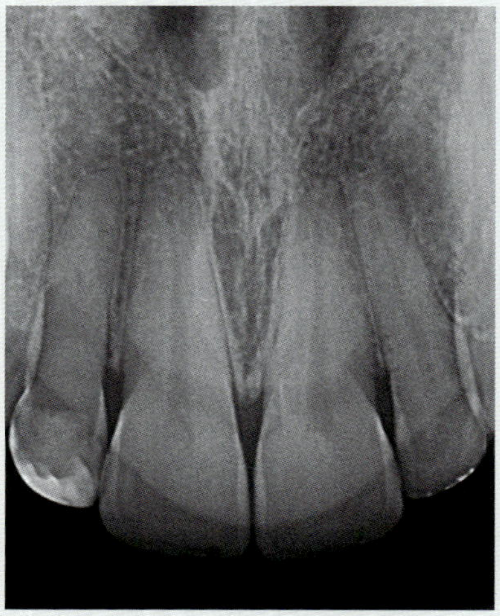

Figure 23 Radiographic check of the restorations 15 years later.

CONCLUSION

Composite nowadays allows the discerning clinician to create aesthetic restorations of excellent quality and minimal invasiveness, with low costs for patients and more than satisfactory results at a distance, especially if with proper maintenance performed with simple re-polishing procedures.

The margin of risk of our work over time is also reduced: we can re-intervene with relative ease in the management of fractures or defects that might show up over the years, repairing without necessarily redoing the restorations from scratch, with conservative and economic advantages for our patients. The concerns for many clinicians in approaching these materials are related to chairside time and the complexity in achieving an aesthetic result that can be appreciated on a daily basis, so more invasive techniques such as ceramic restorations are sometimes preferred. The authors believe that working times are inevitably linked to certain unavoidable steps (preparation, adhesive phase, apposition of limited amounts of composite to reduce the shrinkage phenomenon, polymerization with adequate timing of each layer of material), and that a correctly approached layering technique, using the available tools and guides presented in this contribution, provides the clinician with the key to achieve a clinical and aesthetic success appreciable for a long time.

SUGGESTED READINGS

- Devoto W. Clinical procedures for producing aesthetic stratified composite resin restorations. *Pract Proced Aesthet Dent.* 2002;14(7):541-544.
- Devoto W, Pansecchi D. Composite restorations in the anterior region: clinical and aesthetic performances. *Pract Proced Aesthet Dent.* 2007;19(8):465-470.
- Devoto W, Saracinelli M, Manauta J. Composite in everyday practice: How to choose the right material and simplify techniques in the anterior teeth. *Eur J Esthet Dent.* 2010;5(1):102-24.
- Devoto W, Vanini L. Rifinitura e lucidatura dei restauri in composito. *Il Dentista Moderno*, Dossier, 5-13, 1999.
- Manauta J, Salat A, Monterubbianesi R et al. Advances in diastema closure and tooth shape change using direct composite restorations: the Front Wing Technique. *Int J Esthet Dent.* 2022;17(4):378-393.
- Monteiro P. The step by step in finishing and polishing anterior direct composite restorations. *Styleitaliano.org.* 2017.
- Villares CF. Diastema closure a single shade opacity aesthetic approach. *Styleitaliano.org.* 2019.

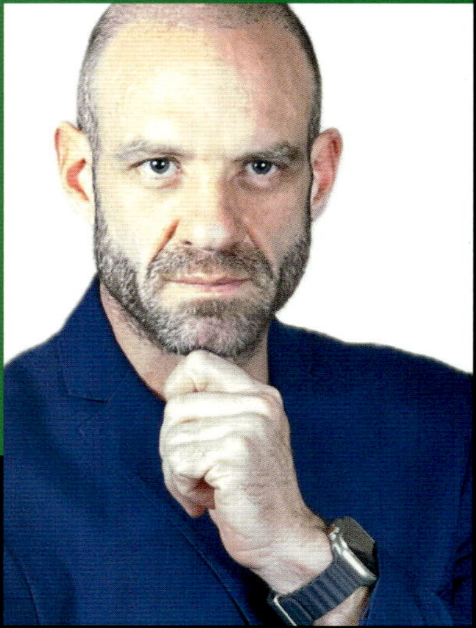

JORDI MANAUTA

Mexico, Italy

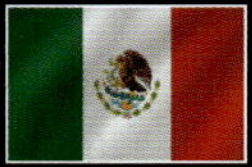

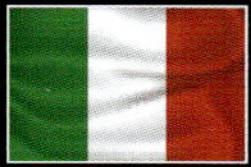

Jordi Manauta was born in Mexico City. He graduated with honors from the Technological University of Mexico (UNITEC). He earned a Master's degree in Operative and Aesthetic Dentistry from the International University of Catalonia (UIC) in Barcelona.
In 2022, he was appointed Honorary Professor at the University of Buenos Aires and, in 2024, Global Community Professor at the University of Monterrey in Nuevo Leon, Mexico (UDEM).
Under the mentorship of Miguel Tames (Mexico) and Walter Devoto (Italy), he played a pioneering role in advanced aesthetic dentistry. He is renowned for designing and inventing numerous cutting-edge dental instruments and materials, thanks to collaborations with international companies.
He serves as a scientific consultant for two prestigious European journals, and he has been an active member of StyleItaliano since 2008 and the Italian Society of Conservative Dentistry (SIDOC).
As a speaker at courses and conferences, he is the author and co-author of several publications in international scientific journals.

SEMI-DIRECT VENEERS, REALISTIC TRY-IN AND COMPLEX COLOR VALIDATION

Color matching with direct composites has been one of the strongest challenges in aesthetic dentistry, especially when talking about single central restorations, as in a Class IV or a unitary veneer. It is important to highlight that in our philosophy before the restoration is built, color matching has 2 mandatory stages, color evaluation and color validation.

COLOR EVALUATION

A first approach to color, gives the clinician the first notion of what material color or colors we must use for the tooth we want to restore, classically this is done with a commercial shade guide (1), system oriented shade guides (2), personalized shade guides (3),

Figure 1 Commercial shade guides, provide a fair color estimation, it is unclear how the clinician should interpret and select materials of the color obtained and are skill dependent.

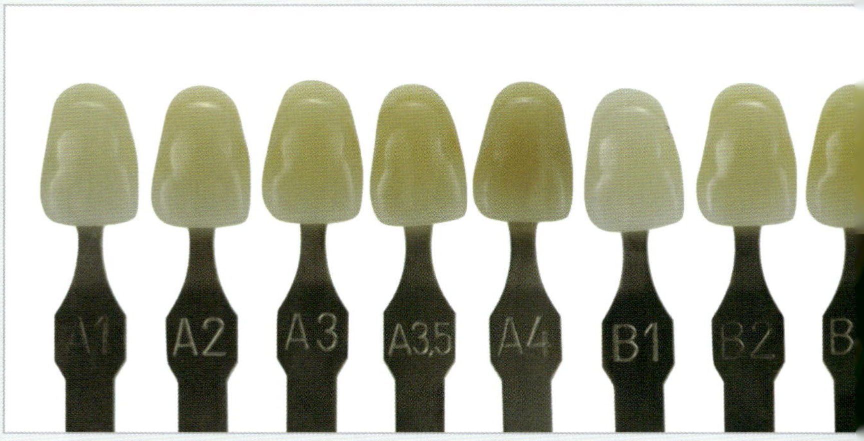

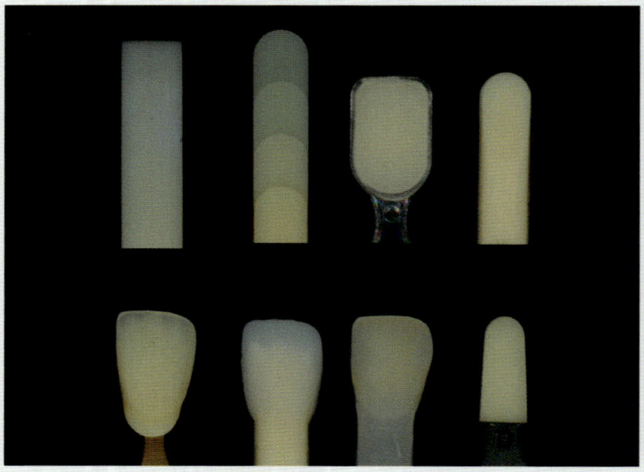

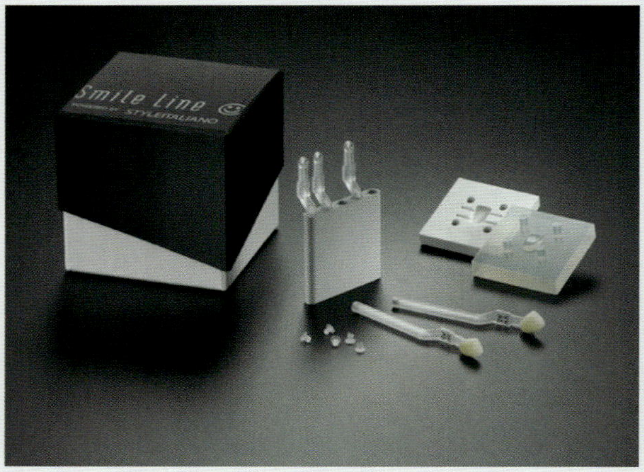

Figure 2 System based shade guides, although suggested by each manufacturer as the best option, recent evidence has shown that the color correspondence of the shade guide with the actual restorative material is poor and sometimes entirely inaccurate, often becoming more misleading than helpful information.

Figure 3 Personalized shade guide allows the user to self-fabricate single or dual shade-guide tabs with the actual material that will be used for the final restoration. This is one of the most reliable methods and it is always suggested to have available.

and digital colorimeters compatible with layering app/software (**📷 4**), even if all of the work with certain reliability, the latter have proven to be the most accurate.
Whichever color evaluation method is used, it is mandatory to validate the colors selected, this brings us to the next stage.

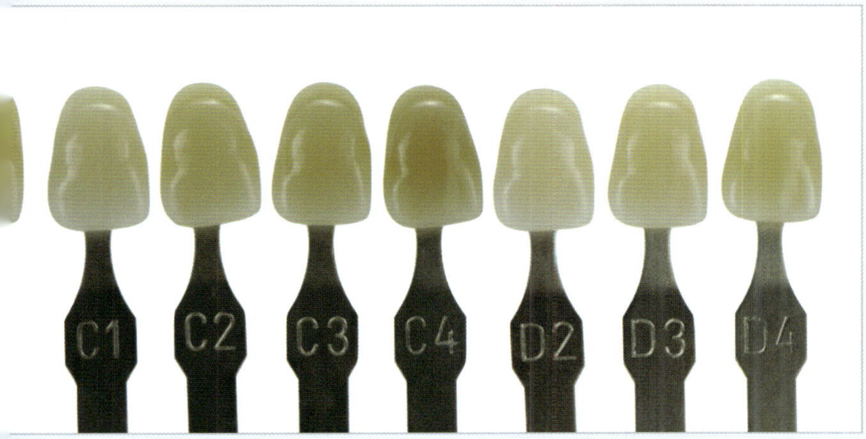

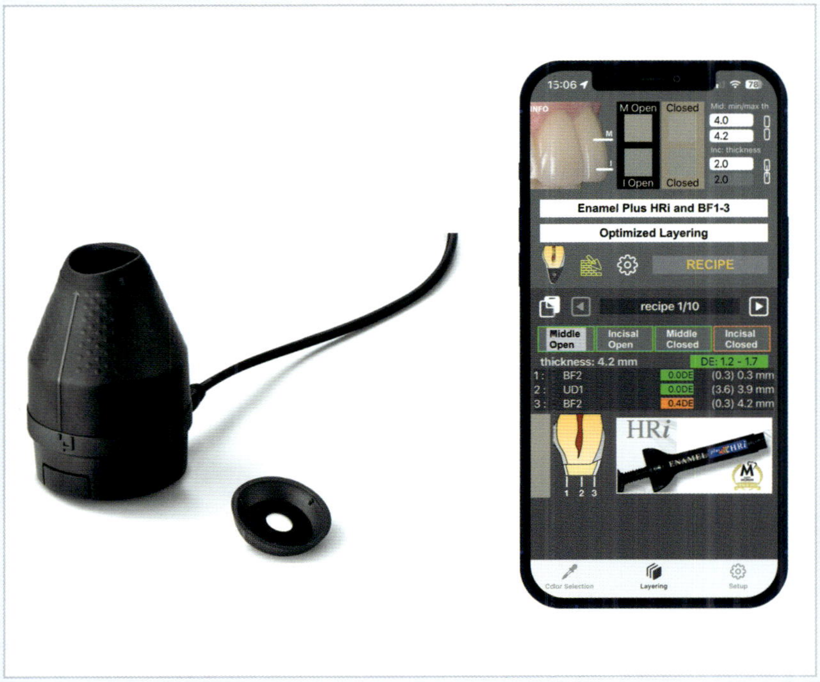

Figure 4 New generation colorimeters (Optishade, Smile Line) managed by smartphone/tablets are equipped with apps that are able to calculate composite recipes (Compashade, Micerium) and predict with much accuracy layering recipes to match the color of a layered restoration.

COLOR VALIDATION

Validating a color requires the restoration to have an acceptable integration in the mouth, under common and normal conditions, judged by veracious observers (at least, patient and clinician). This can represent an enormous challenge, but there are several ways to do it:

A. Final restoration
B. Button try-in
C. Realistic try-in.

A. Final restoration is not a very reliable way to validate your selected colors, it is not immediate, and if something goes wrong, the full restoration has to be re-done, risking time loss and discomfort to the patient. It is strongly recommended not to do final restorations without being sure about the outcome.

B. The button try-in, which is probably the most popular try-in method, is done by placing small amounts of composite in the surface of the opposite tooth to be restored, and it is logically one of the most widespread techniques because of the ease to its accessibility, all that is needed is the actual composite.
It has three main disadvantages. First, the masses used for the try-in suffer a strong

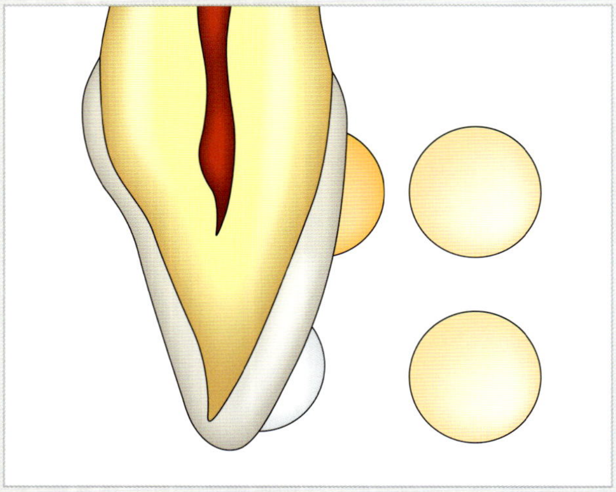

Figure 5 Depiction of the blending effect of the aesthetic materials during the button try-in. The buttons in the right are supposed to be an A2 color, the same composite when connected to the natural tooth will "absorb" the color of the different parts of the tooth (cervical and incisal), changing drastically their appearance.

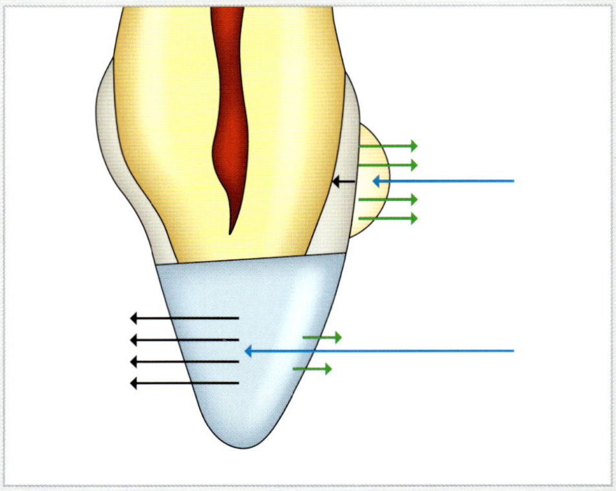

Figure 6 The button that lies on top of the healthy tooth structure will reflect more light and will have a whiter appearance, the same composite in a see-trough cavity (Class IV) will absorb more light and will appear gray despite the good appearance of the button over the healthy tooth.

blending effect **(📷 5)** with the underlying healthy tissues and with the surrounding environment, this happens because the composite samples are very thin and it gives an altered perceived color, in other words, the small button applied to the tooth gets the aspect of the healthy tooth **(📷 6)**. It allows only single shade trials, even if multiple shades are used, they are only seen individually in the surface.

C. The realistic try-in, proposed by the authors in the book *Layers 2* 2022, it is intended to simulate with the actual materials the final restoration, but in the color matching stage, without bonding the restoration.

The purpose of this strategy is to recreate as much as possible the conditions of the final restoration. Same position, same context, same masses, same thicknesses and same shape over the real hydrated tooth and over the already prepared margin free of contaminants **(📷 7-11)**.

After achieving this, we will have the best available preview. There is no other better color validation method that we know. Often, the desired color is not found on a composite system, suggesting to the clinician to switch system, making it incredibly valuable information.

It allows multi shade try-in, by overlapping and simulating the stratification

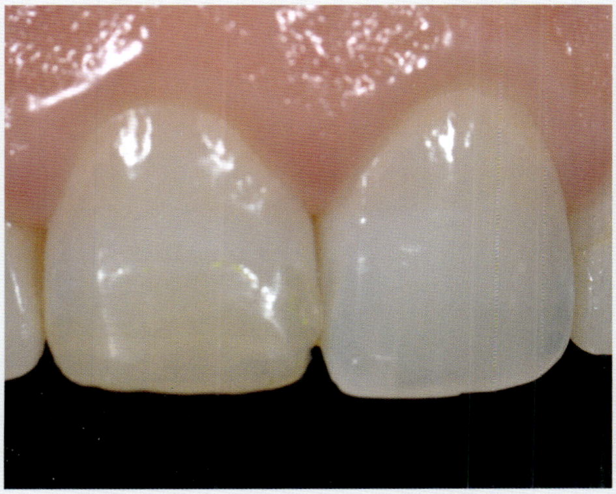

Figure 7 A defective Class IV restoration to be replaced, it represents one of the most difficult challenges in esthetic restorative dentistry.

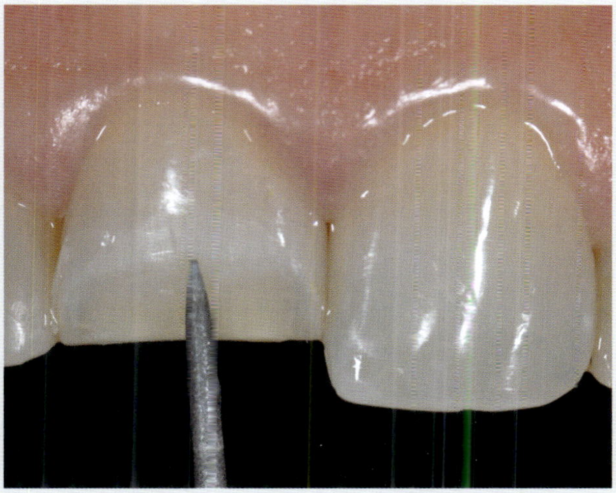

Figure 8 To perform a successful realistic try-in it is mandatory to recreate the final situation as closely as possible. This is achievable by removing the old restoration and already creating the final margin/bevel, paying attention not to dehydrate the tooth.

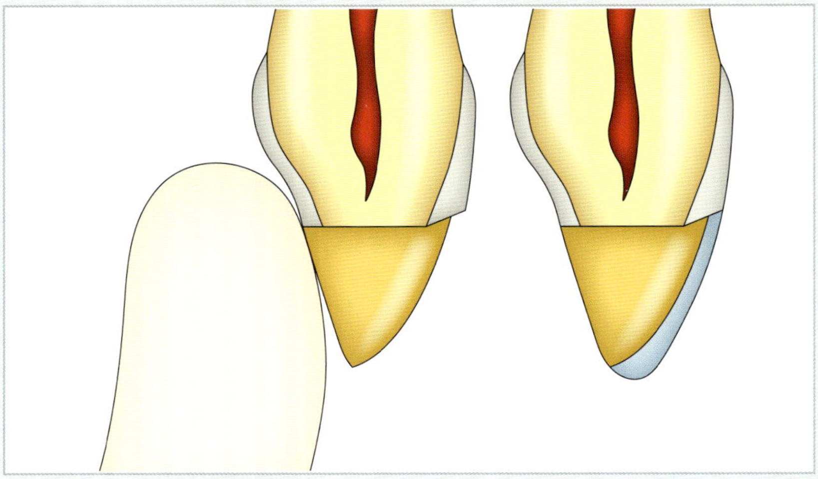

Figure 9 Without etching or bonding, a layer of dentin is placed and polymerized, a surface layer (enamel) is placed on top, these two masses will recreate the basic color of the tooth.

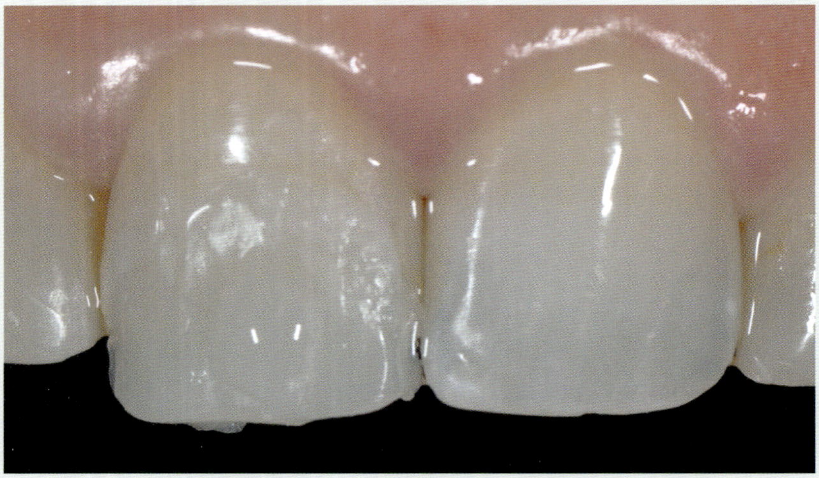

Figure 10 The dentin/enamel non bonded try-in is evaluated inside the mouth, in the real place, with the real thicknesses and with the actual materials that will be used in the restoration. If the try-in looks good the recipe will be replicated, if on the contrary the try-in looks bad, a second try-in will be done taking into consideration the previous information. With this information the recipe for performing the final restoration can be improved.

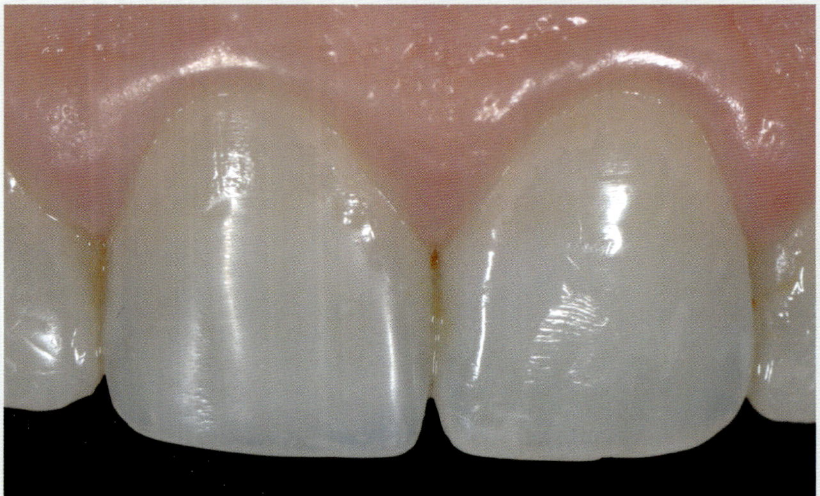

Figure 11 The final restoration done with the same recipe that was obtained during the realistic try-in. The restoration was further improved with characterizations in the incisal third.

The possibilities related to the "realistic try-in" try method are very advantageous. They are all quite intuitive, yet, listing them is important to get a broad understanding of the possible direct workflows you will find in this book.

- As mentioned before, the realistic try-in allows for the most precise direct color matching, as it is done with the same composite of our system, in that very context and hydration, with an almost exact thickness and shape.
- Although it requires good experience with anterior restorations to reproduce the mock-up in the final restoration, it allows for a multi-shade matching.
- It is a very effective strategy for the fabrication of a silicone index.
- It allows for immediate occlusion check, which is especially useful when restoring worn anterior teeth.
- When convenient, it may be part of a semi-direct restoration strategy.
- Mastering the realistic try-in often brings superb pre-restorations, these, when detached is possible to make small corrections, cement them as a final restoration.

SEMI-DIRECT RESTORATIONS

Securing a successful realistic try-in gives us not only precious information, but already a true physical restoration, if this unbounded restoration can be safely removed, it can still be perfection, by finishing it, adding-on, relining or trimming.

This semi-direct technique relies on all the advantages of a direct restoration, such as a realistic try-in immediate color assessment and marginal precision and as if this weren't already enough, it has all the advantages of an indirect technique, such as the possibility of post-polymerization, extra-oral finishing and relining.

Originally described in the '80s for posterior inlays, this approach is today applied in many situations, such as in composite veneer restorations, as recently described by Newton Fahl Jr. in his book *Composite Veneers: The Direct-Indirect Technique*, and who is probably the world's most expert exponent in this topic. Some complex unitary cases are published in the book *Layers 2* by the authors of the article.

Clinical case

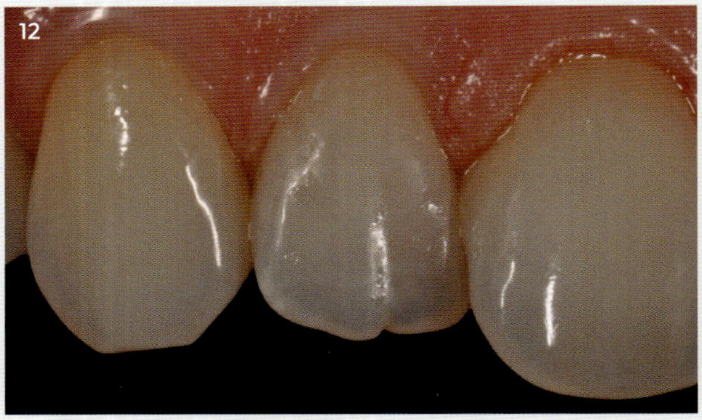

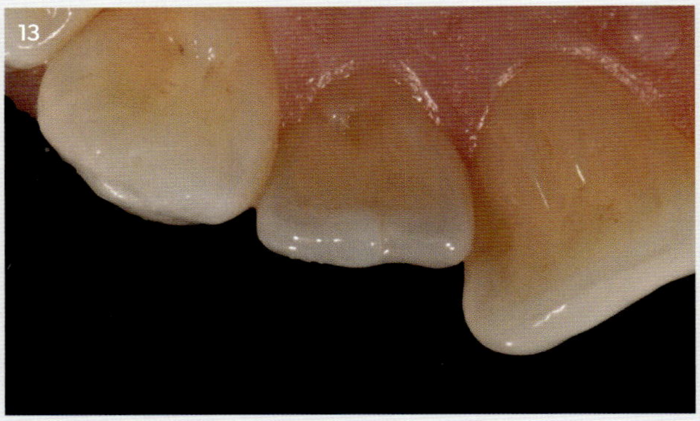

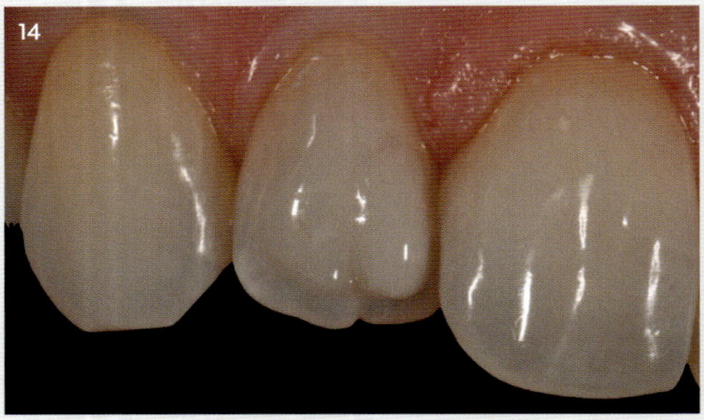

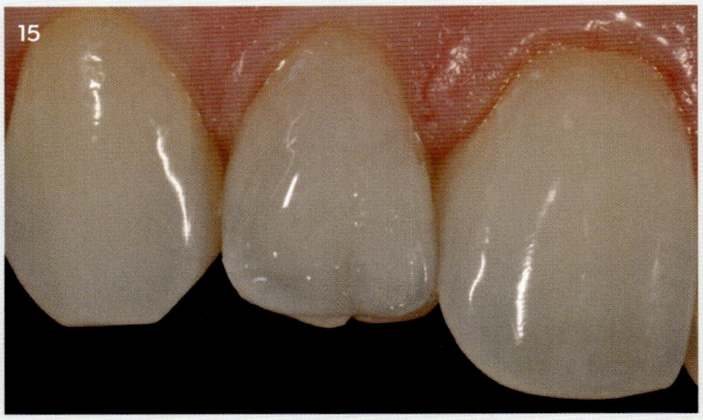

Figure 12 Initial situation, a misaligned tooth 1.2 with esthetically unpleasant results for the patient.

Figure 13 Same initial situation from an occlusal view, showing the misalignment and how much space is available to correct the defect additively without the need of prepping or other more invasive alternatives.

Figure 14 A white dentin (UD0,5 Enamel plus HRi, Micerium, Italy) was used to recreate the internal anatomy of the tooth, the dental core was modeled following the external contour of the natural tooth, the dentin was placed with a continuous profile from the cervical, once modeled we polymerized.

Figure 15 Given the good outcome of the dentin we decided to add an opalescent mass in the incisal edge to get a good and natural characterization (OBN, Enamel Plus HFO, Micerium, Italy).

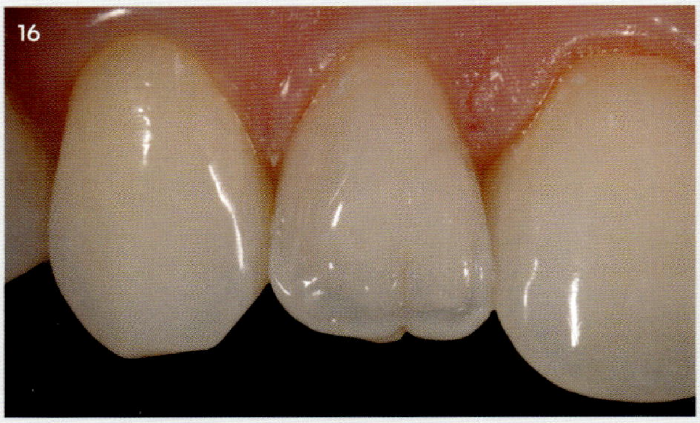

Figure 16 The incisal halo was recreated using an opaque mass, in this case the same dentin used for the core, doing a roll to simulate the counter opalescence opacity (UD0,5, Enamel Plus HRi, Micerium, Italy). All this process was done fairly quickly to avoid dehydration of the teeth.

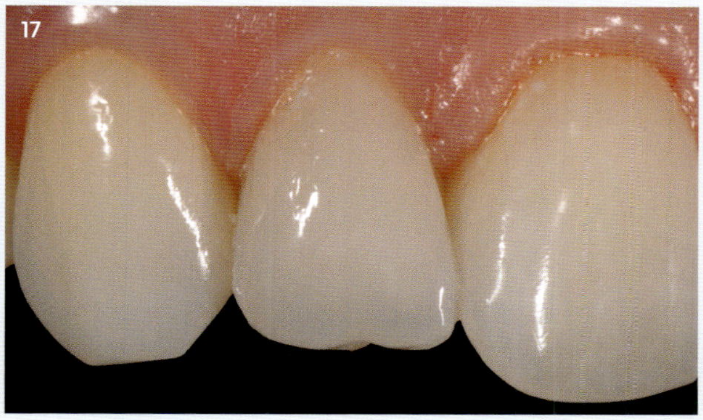

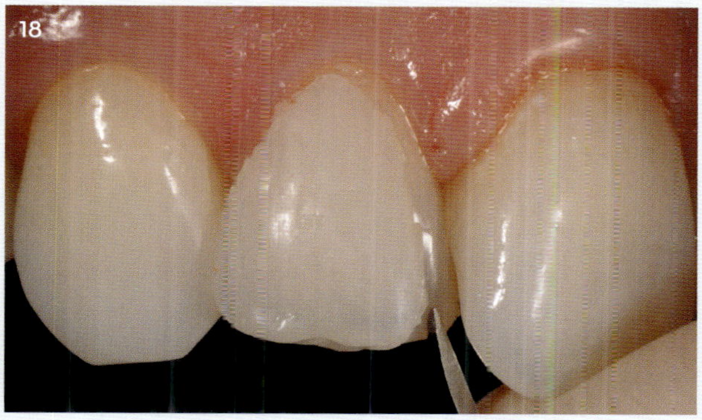

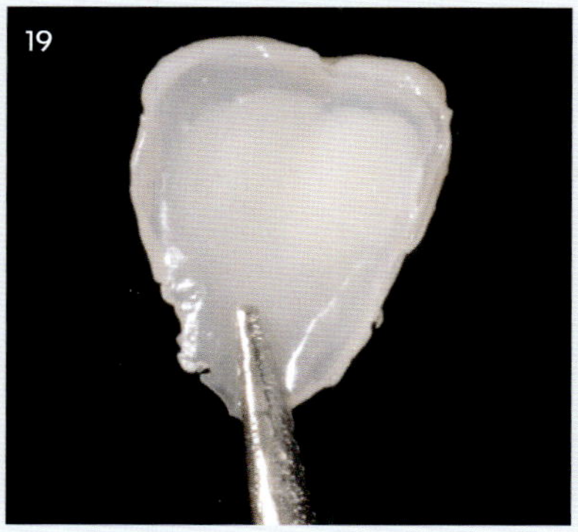

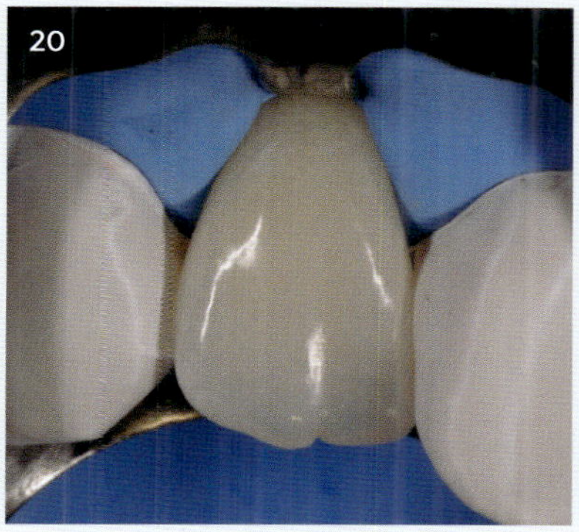

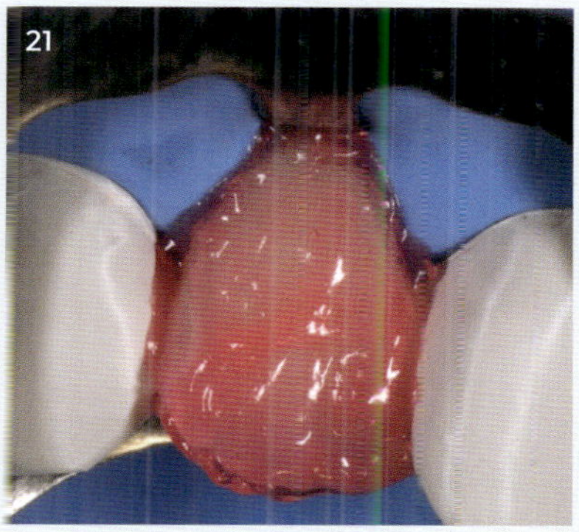

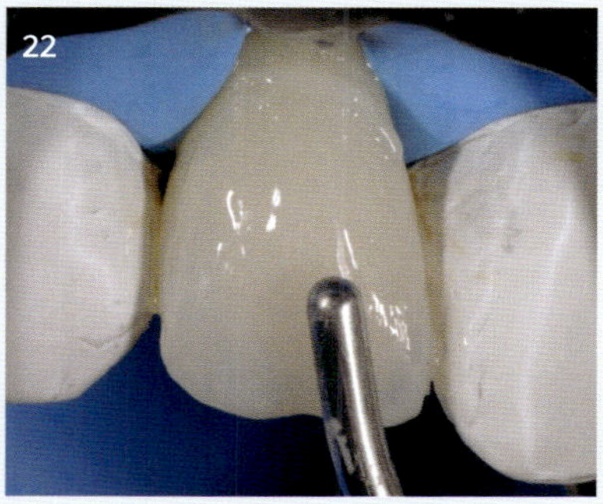

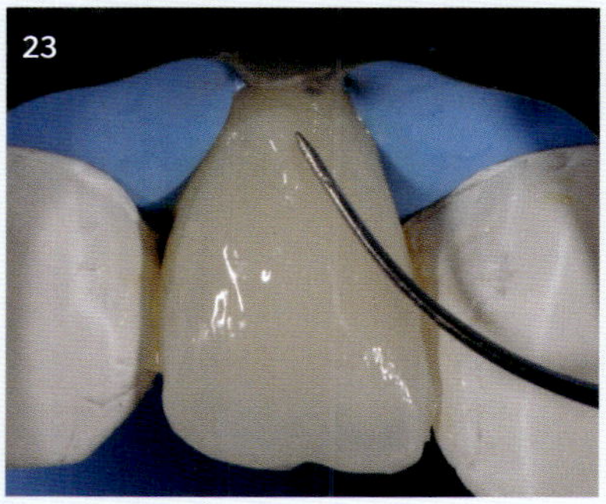

Figure 17 The final layer was done with a high value enamel (UE3 Enamel Plus HRi, Micerium, Italy) and thoroughly polymerized. The patient was left undisturbed and the teeth under the moisture of the saliva. After some minutes, together with the patient, we assessed the aspect of the restoration, which appeared absolutely perfect.

Figure 18 The next step is the detachment of the realistic try-in, normally, if there are no undercuts, the restoration is very easy to remove and it requires no previous lubricants or separators, it should come in one unique piece.

Figure 19 The detached piece held with delicate tweezers. With the help of an abrasive disk, we will be able to remove overhanging material and marginal imperfections. It is advised to work inside a container, with magnification and holding delicately with the fingers because the restoration could inadvertently fall.

Figure 20 The tooth is isolated and the adjacent teeth protected from etching. An extra try-in is done to ensure there are no obstacles for the final fitting during the cementation stage.

Figure 21 Acid etching of the enamel and the subsequent application of a universal bonding agent.

Figure 22 The semi-direct restoration was cemented with a transparent Veneer cement (RelyX Veneers, 3M, USA), we prefer photo cured materials which allow a very small film thickness but that allow enough consistency for a comfortable excess removal.

Figure 23 Excess removal with Fissura instrument (LM Arte, LM Dental, Finland) and afterwards with Compobrush (Smile Line, Switzerland).

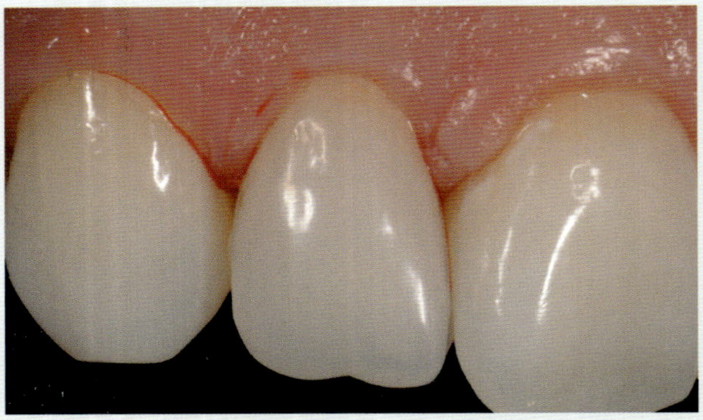

Figure 24 After final polymerization a quick finishing and polishing was performed and the tuber dam was removed. We cannot evaluate the color at this stage, neither positively nor negatively. In other words, if the restoration looks too dark or too white, we must wait until gingival tissues are back to normal and the dental structures are rehydrated again.

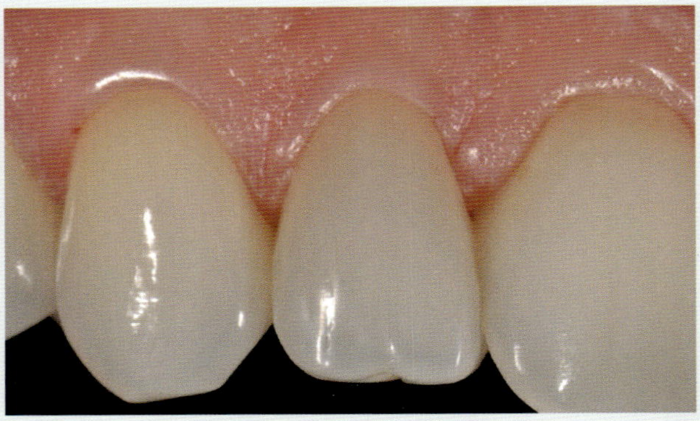

Figure 25 Follow-up after one week, we can see how good the integration is: now any color defect can be properly addressed, but this is very unlikely to happen as we saw the final outcome before starting the restoration.

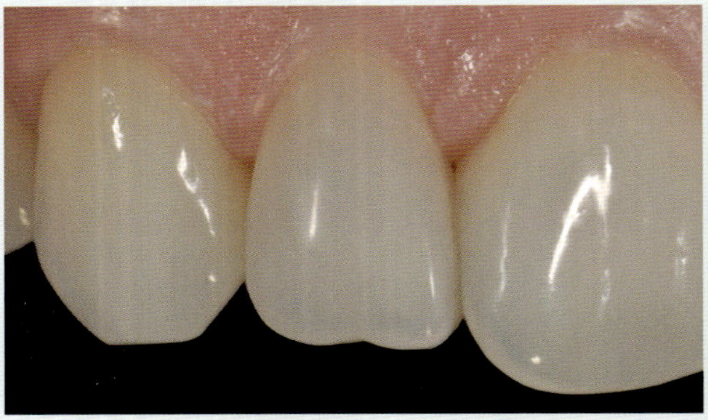

Figure 26 Follow-up after 1 year.

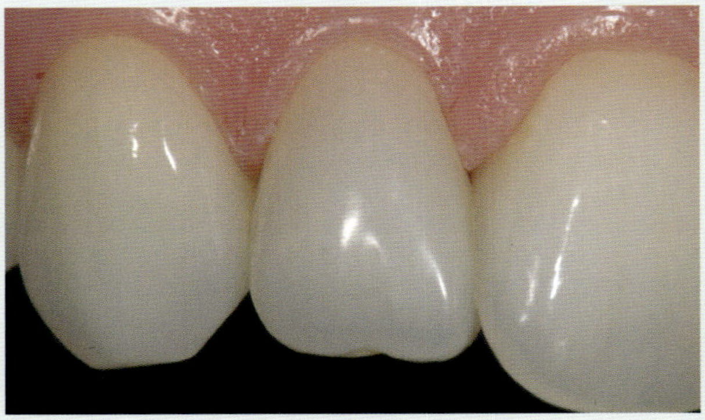

Figure 27 Follow-up after 4 years.

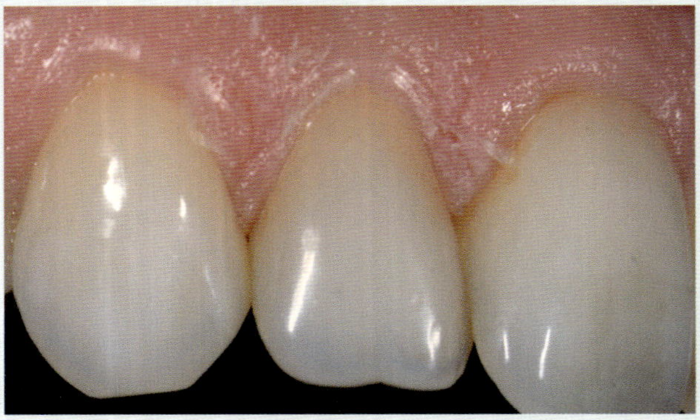

Figure 28 Follow-up after 7 years.

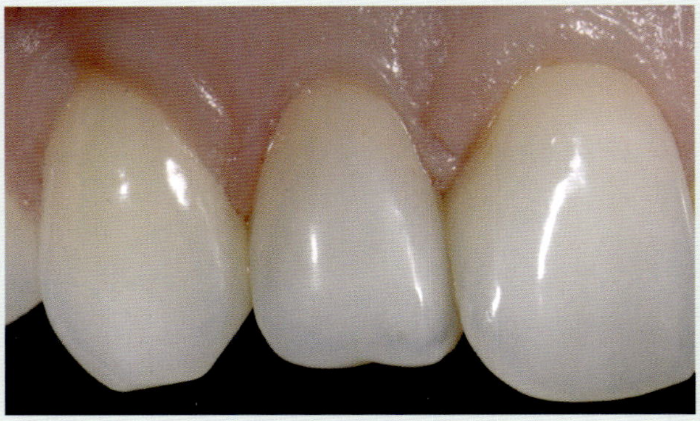

Figure 29 Follow-up after 10 years.

CONCLUSION

There is no other better color matching method than seeing the real restoration in the context of the normality of the patient's mouth. With the different color evaluation methods, the digital ones being the most accurate, we can opt for a realistic try-in to validate our findings, no matter which one we choose. Commonly the realistic try-in is already an outstanding restoration that with little post-production can become a restoration that we can cement, with the certainty that the color will be perfect.

In short, digital colorimetry with layering predictions is the optimal evaluation method for color, the realistic try-in is the most accurate validation method, and the semi-direct (direct-indirect) technique can help make all of this a reality.

SUGGESTED READINGS

- Browning WD, Contreras-Bulnes R, Brackett MG, Brackett WW. Color differences: polymerized composite and corresponding Vitapan Classical shade tab. *J Dent.* 2009;37:34-39.
- Calixto R, Eustaquio J. Direct – *Facetas em resinas compostas.* Santos Publicaçoes, 2021.
- Fahl Jr. N, Ritter A. *Composite Veneers: The direct-Indirect Technique.* Quintessence Publishing, 2020.
- Manauta J, Salat A. *Layers: An atlas of composite resin stratification.* Quintessence Publishing, 2012.
- Manauta J, Salat A, Devoto W, Putignano A. *Layers 2: The Styelitaliano clinical secrets.* Quintessence Publishing, 2022.
- Manauta J, Salat A, Putignano A et al. Stratification in anterior teeth using one dentine shade and a predefined thickness of enamel: a new concept in composite layering – Part I. *Odontostomatol Trop.* 2014;37(146):5-16.
- Manauta J, Salat A, Putignano A et al. Stratification in anterior teeth using one dentine shade and a predefined thickness of enamel: a new concept in composite layering – Part 2. *Odontostomatol Trop.* 2014;37(147) 5-13.
- Miller L. Organizing color in dentistry. *J Am Dent Assoc.* 1987;Spec No:26E-40E.
- Paravina RD, Westland S, Imai FH et al. Evaluation of blending effect of composites related to restoration size. *Dent Mater.* 2006;22(4):299-307.
- Rizzi A, Bonanomi C, Brazzoli S et al. Assessing appearance in human dental colour space. *Computer Methods in Biomechanics and Biomedical Engineering: Imaging & Visualization.* 2016;6(1):59-67.

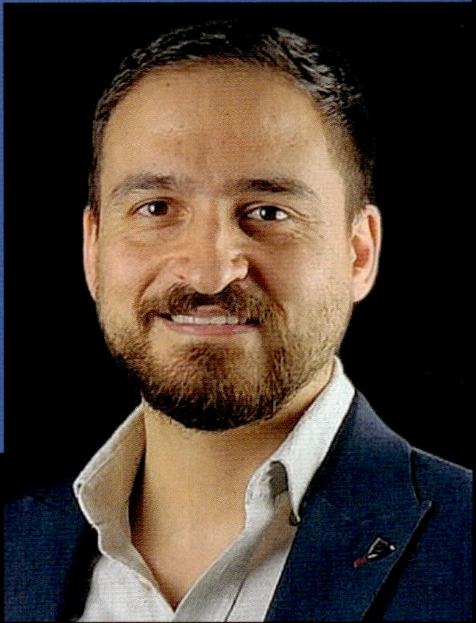

MAROUN GHALEB

Lebanon

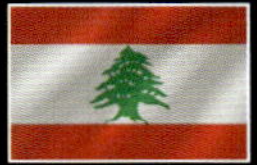

Maroun Ghaleb obtained his degree in Dental Surgery in 2012 and his Master's degree in Prosthetic and Aesthetic Dentistry in 2015 from Saint Joseph University of Beirut. Since then, he has been a lecturer at the same university in the Department of Restorative and Aesthetic Dentistry for preclinical and clinical courses.

A specialist in aesthetic and prosthetic dentistry, he is the inventor of the MOOS technique, published in 2017 on StyleItaliano website, of which he is an active member.

Actively involved in research, he has published numerous articles in international journals and given lectures and workshops on direct composite veneers.

He runs a private practice in Lebanon, focusing on direct anterior

VESTIBULAR INDEX TECHNIQUE: A NOVEL APPROACH SIMPLIFYING DIRECT VENEERING

Direct composite veneers are a successful and highly aesthetic treatment, but hold several challenges that complicate the clinical procedure and impact the final outcome. The major challenge is related to the corrections needed, requiring more than one session to achieve clinical success. This can be explained by the absence of a clear reference driving the veneering process. As a matter of fact, not initially following a reference can jeopardize the aesthetic outcome by increasing the risk of having disproportioned teeth, tilted or shifted midline and bulky restorations. In addition, obtaining the optimal buccal contour of the teeth is a crucial aesthetic parameter, and if the latter is not defined from the beginning, finishing time is maximized by having more excess material going to waste. This also compromises the final layering by removing layers of composite to correct the buccal contour.
Another thing that can be tricky with composite veneers is the "surprise effect". Patients don't see the final result until the end of the treatment, which can sometimes lead to them rejecting the design and requiring rework. Overcoming these difficult challenges is now possible with this novel approach called: The Vestibular Index technique. In this article, a detailed step by step protocol of this technique is presented in a case of eight anterior composite veneers.

DISCUSSION AND CLINICAL CASE

A 28-year-old man presented to our clinic complaining of his anterior teeth aesthetics. He had two Emax crowns on teeth 21 and 22 because of past trauma. The centrals are neither proportional nor symmetrical. His canines and his left premolar are in a palatal position and are barely visible when smiling. The laterals are rotated distally and the two crowns are bulkier than the adjacent teeth **(📷 1-4)**.

The patient wanted a whiter color for his final restorations and wished to restore the incisal edges.

The initial treatment plan was to start with an orthodontic treatment to correct the alignment, followed by aesthetic restoration of the anterior teeth by doing a gingivectomy for

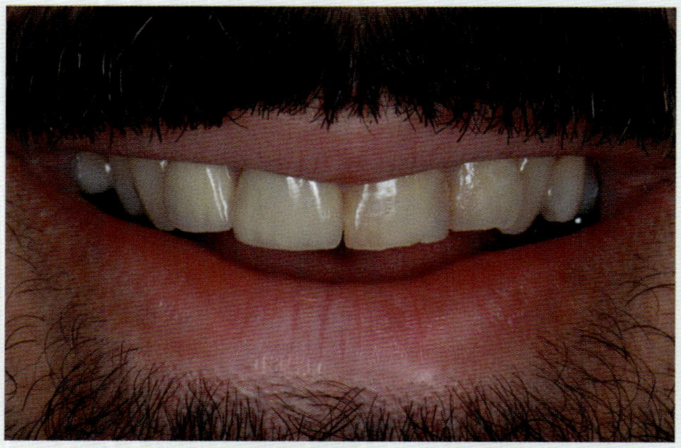

Figure 1 Preoperative extraoral front picture.

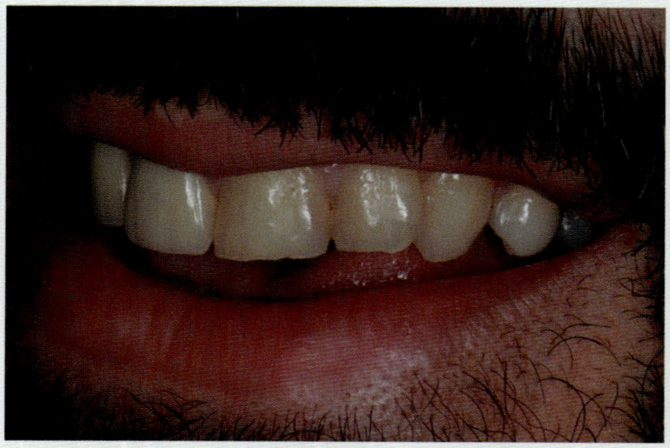

Figure 2 Preoperative right view.

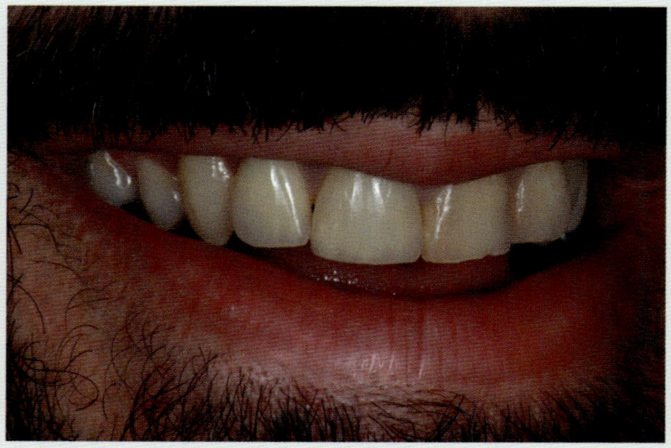

Figure 3 Preoperative left view.

the centrals to correct the gingival level, two new crowns on teeth 21 and 22 along with two veneers on teeth 11 and 12. Bleaching was suggested to whiten the teeth and obtain a brighter smile. The patient refused this plan because it was out of his budget, it would take time to be achieved and he had a private event coming up. That's why eight anterior composite veneers with bleaching for the lower teeth was proposed as an alternative treatment plan. Diagnostic wax-up can be done either manually (with wax or composite). or digitally. It is important to well define on the wax-up the interproximal areas, transitional lines, smile line and alignment of the teeth (📷 5). A wax-up should always be followed by a clinical mock-up to validate the new parameters if suitable for the patient or not.

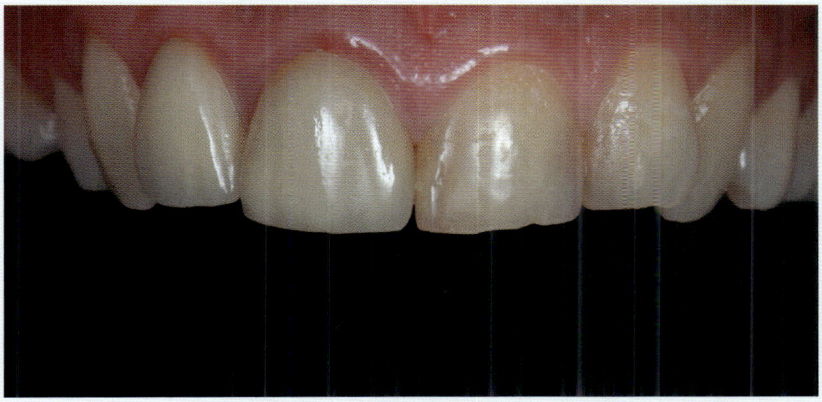

Figure 4 Intraoral view.

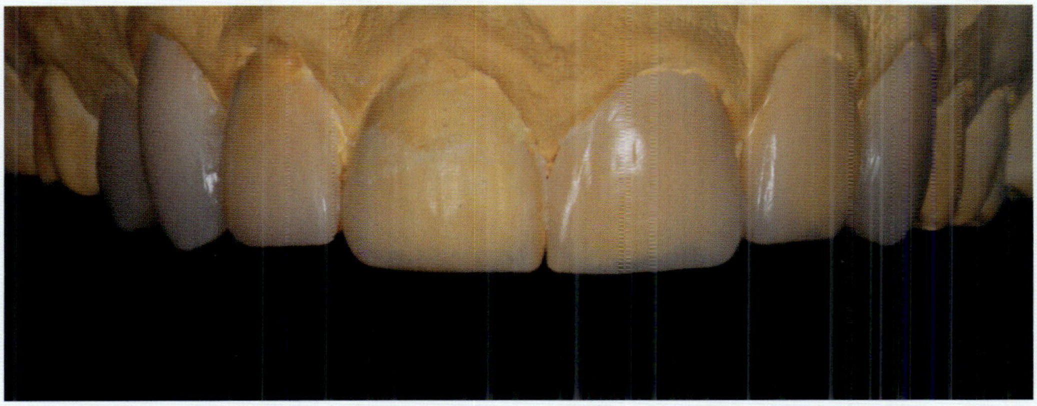

Figure 5 Manual wax-up.

Mock-up special considerations

- Small preparation of teeth 21, 22 and disto-buccal side of the laterals to ensure a perfect placement of the silicone index and enough thickness of resin material.
- Never put anesthesia at this stage. We should be able to evaluate the length and the buccal contour of the teeth without altering the lip position.
- Spot bond should be applied in the middle of the teeth to fix the mock-up in place.
- It is crucial to apply a lubricant (e.g., Vaseline) in the interproximal and palatal areas to prevent adherence of the resin material to the teeth and to facilitate the cutting and the separation of the product later on.
- The silicone index is filled buccally with Luxatemp Star composite resin (DMG), then applied to the teeth until it is completely set. Using a probe, excess material in the cervical area is removed before the final setting (📷 6).
- At this stage of the diagnostic approach, the new volume of the teeth must be approved by the patient, resulting in total agreement on the definition of tooth shape, size and length. We can add or remove from the mock-up until we have total satisfaction and validation of the final design (📷 7).

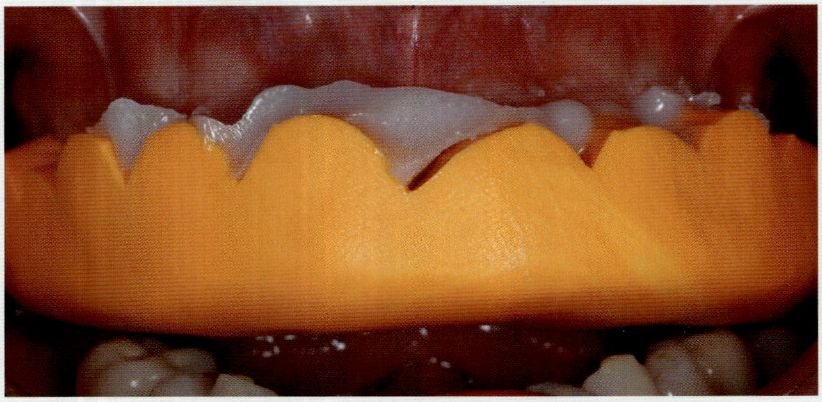

Figure 6 Silicone index filled with Luxatemp Star resin (DMG).

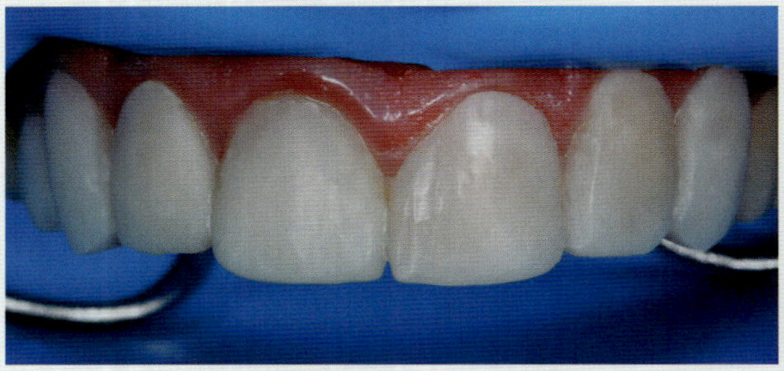

Figure 7 Intraoral view of the mock-up after corrections and polishing.

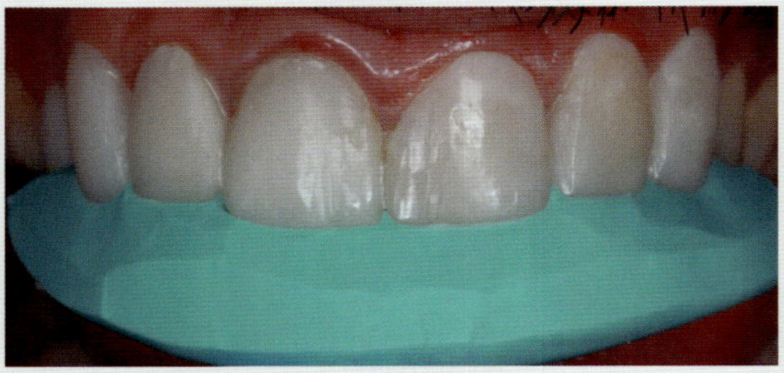

Figure 8 Palatal silicone index.

A palatal index is fabricated using silicone material to record the final incisal edge position (📷 8). This guide does not give us the needed references to restore the buccal contour, that's why in some cases, it is not enough to use it alone.

The Vestibular Index technique is based on using the mock-up to drive the restorative procedure. This has several advantages:

- Reducing the risk of errors and corrections by acting as a physical 3D guide during the restoration of every tooth.
- Guiding the preparation of the teeth (preparation through the mock-up to ensure 0.8 mm for composite material) (📷 9).
- Guaranteeing a perfect proportion between teeth by giving the needed mesio-distal width to reconstruct each tooth (📷 10).
- Reconstructing the axes of the teeth and the midline in a correct way, parallel to the adjacent teeth (📷 11). In fact, when the back-to-back matrix technique is used, some failures are still faced such as tilted, asymmetrical or shifted midline.

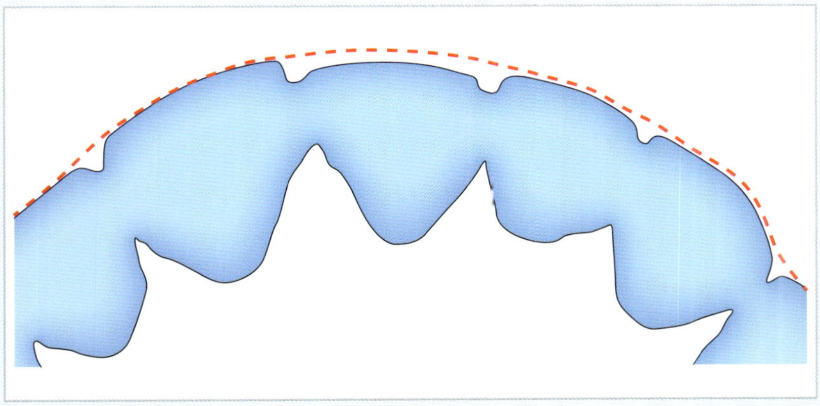

Figure 9

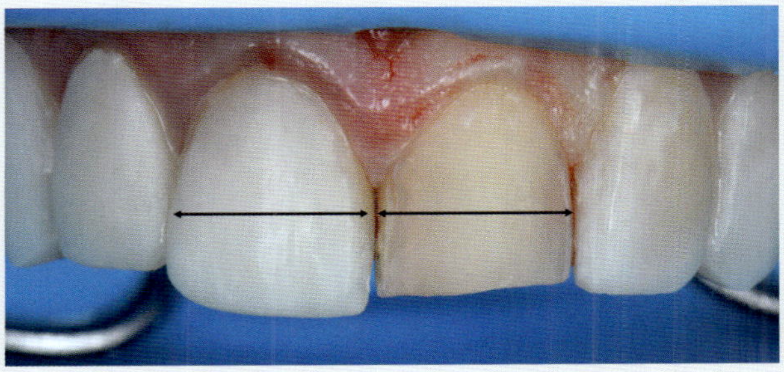

Figure 10

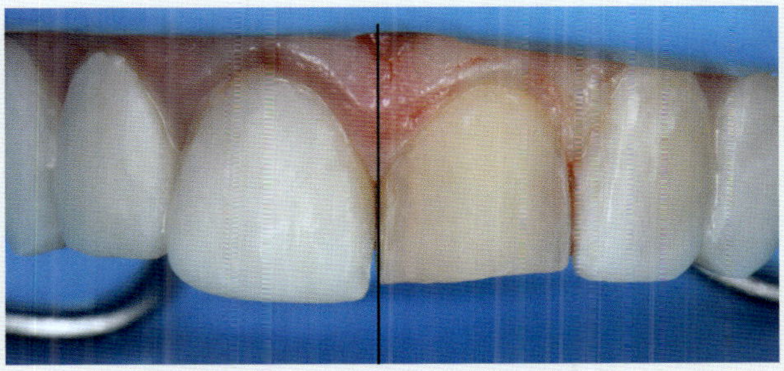

Figure 11

- Reducing the surprise effect: the patient approved on the smile design in the beginning and the final design of the composite veneers will look almost exactly like the mock-up.
- Preserving all the characterizations done in the incisal edge (incisal halo, stains, mamelon). This is due to the precise smile line already obtained from the mock-up.

The preparation of the buccal face is mandatory to ensure at least 0.8 mm for the restorative material. A gauge bur can be used to calibrate the amount of removed tissue (see Figure 9).

An orthodontic disc and a thin needle bur are used to cut the interproximal areas of the right central. It is very important to cut according to the mock-up and to preserve the interproximal references of the adjacent teeth **(📷 12-13)**.

After placing the rubber dam, etching of the tooth was carried out with 37% phosphoric acid (Scotchbond, 3M/ESPE, St. Paul, MN, USA), following the total-etch protocol. Afterwards, the adhesive single bond 2 (3M/ESPE, St. Paul, MN, USA) was applied in two consecutive layers, using a microbrush. A 5 second air spray was performed after each layer to evaporate the solvent followed by light curing for 20 seconds.

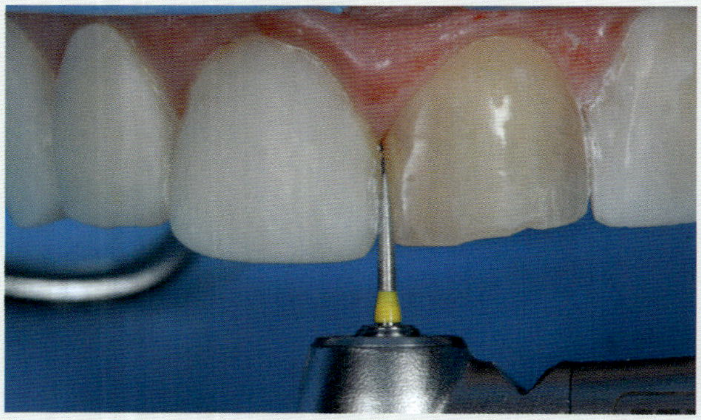

Figure 12

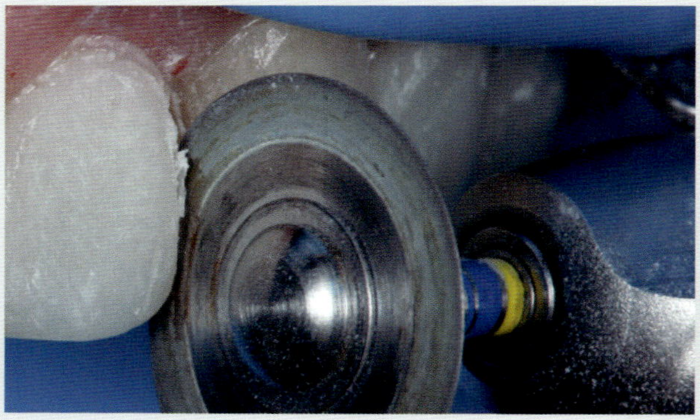

Figure 13

The palatal wall was created by using the palatal index previously done. Si E (CompoSite system from white dental beauty) should always be applied in this part of the tooth (📷 14).
Before Unica matrix placement, it is always better to pass a dental floss between the teeth to make sure that no material is left in the interproximal area that will deform the matrix.
Unica matrix is the ideal matrix to be used with this technique because it helps in building the frame with the right proportions respecting the width of the adjacent central. Its convex proximal surface permits to obtain a rounded contour like the natural teeth. Unica matrix is an anatomical matrix that is designed to conform to the natural anatomy of the tooth and respect the gingival tissue. That's why it can be used without a wedge in most cases. If it is not well adapted to the tooth, it is recommended to place a wedge or liquid dam. In the cervical area, it ensures a closed box where composite can be applied without any fluid leakage from the sulcus (📷 15).
The outer frame was reconstructed in one shot using Si0.5 (CompoSite system from white dental beauty) with a thickness not exceeding 1 mm (📷 16).

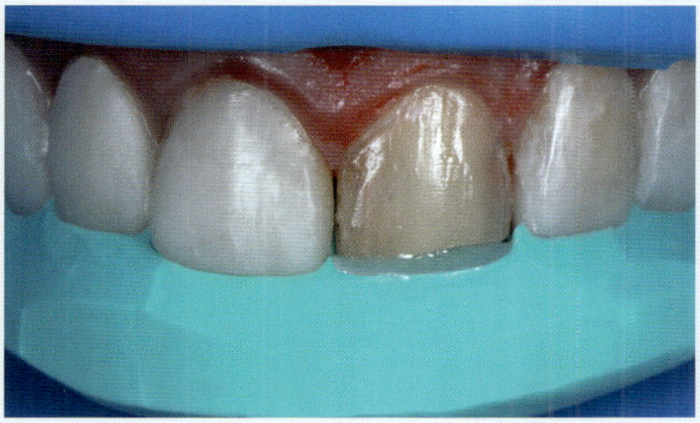

Figure 14

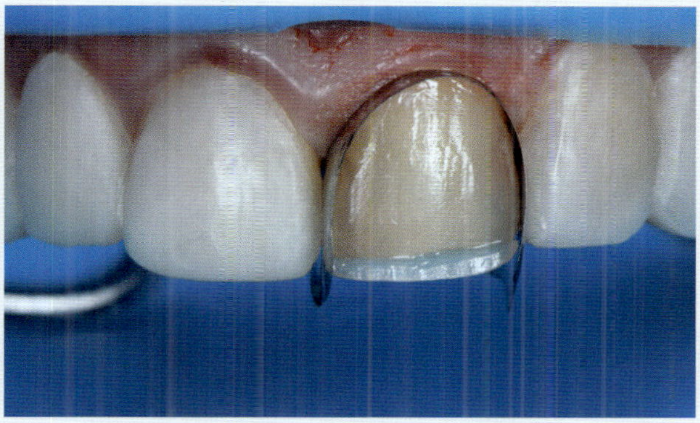

Figure 15

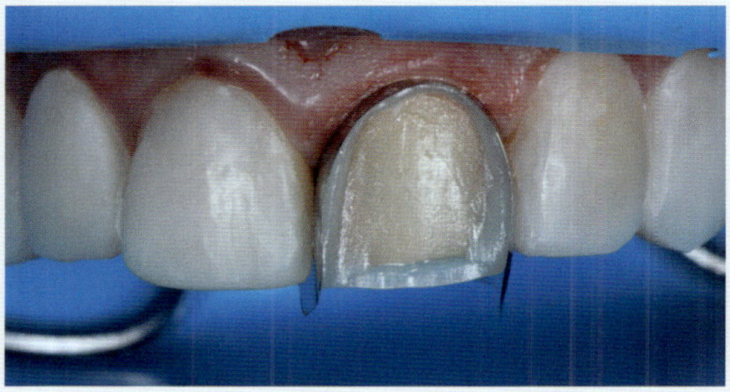

Figure 16

When reconstructing the frame, the mesial wall should be at the same level than that of the adjacent central. The distal wall can be slightly more buccal than the mesial wall of the lateral **(📷 17)**.
If an excess of material is noticed, it is better to remove it with a bur or Sof-Lex disc before proceeding to the buccal part in order to preserve the buccal contour already defined in the mock-up step.
Perfect proportions between the two centrals can be noticed. The dimensions can be measured using a ruler, to double check the width of the teeth. In addition, the axe of the tooth is in concordance with the adjacent teeth. Midline is straight and parallel to the adjacent central **(📷 18)**.

At this stage, two options are feasible:

- Proceed by doing tooth by tooth: this is applicable especially if one shade restorations are done.
- Finish the outer frame of all the teeth, then proceed to the buccal part: it helps in shaping the mamelons at the same time on the anterior teeth to copy them perfectly.

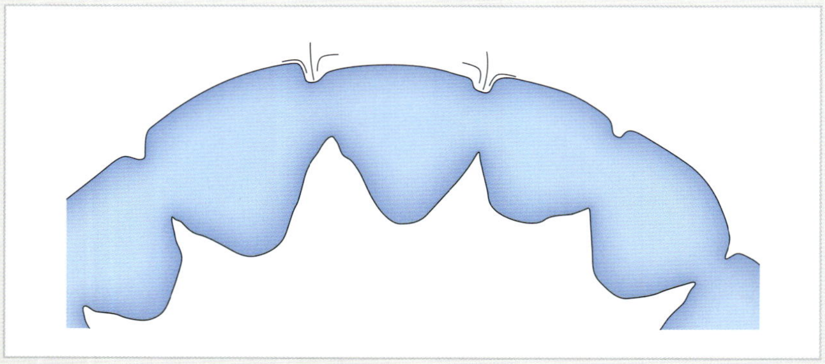

Figure 17

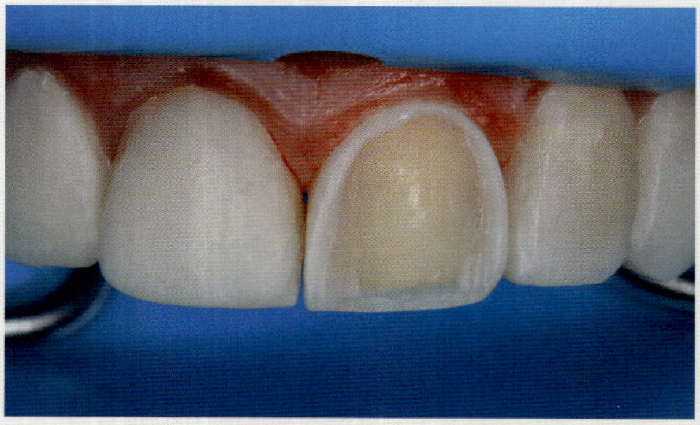

Figure 18

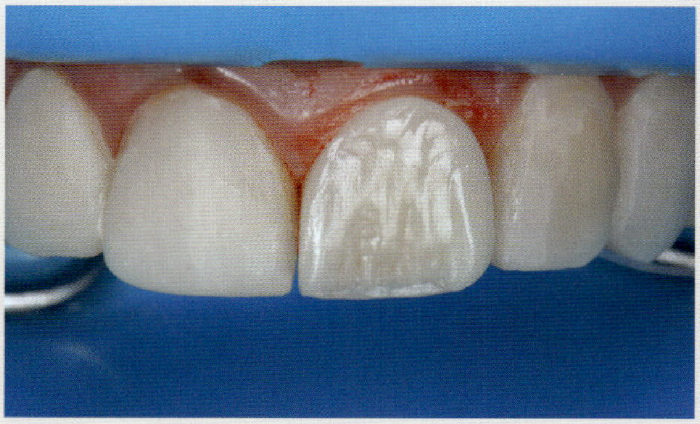

Figure 19

Si 0.5 (CompoSite system from white dental beauty) was applied on the buccal area without exceeding the proximal walls. A 0.5 mm space is left for the final enamel layer (📷 19). Final enamel layer Si E (CompoSite system from white dental beauty) using solo anterior (LM-Dental) was applied (📷 20).

A view from behind the patient is very important to check the final buccal contour. Small corrections must be done to the contour and to the buccal position of the central before progressing to the next one (📷 21).

Restorations

Left central restoration

After finishing the preparation of tooth 21, hydrofluoric acid was applied for 60 seconds to roughen the ceramic's surface. Two layers of silane were carried out followed by the application of the adhesive (📷 22, 23).

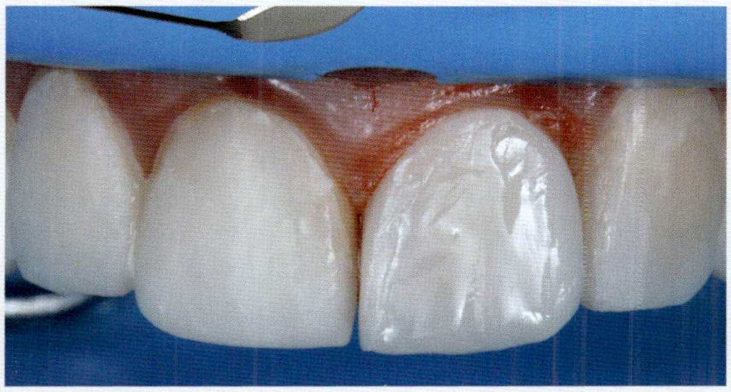

Figure 20

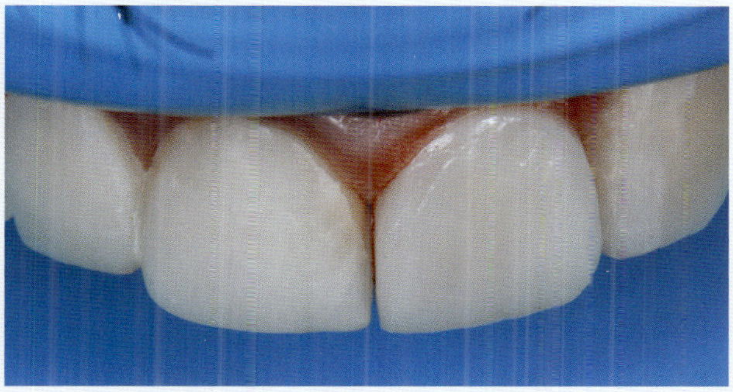

Figure 21

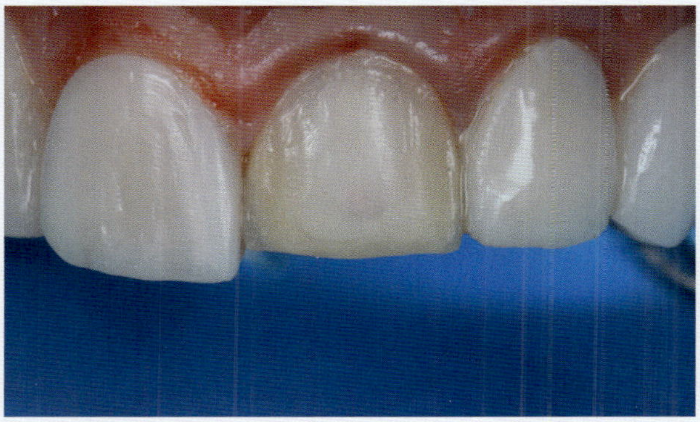

Figure 22

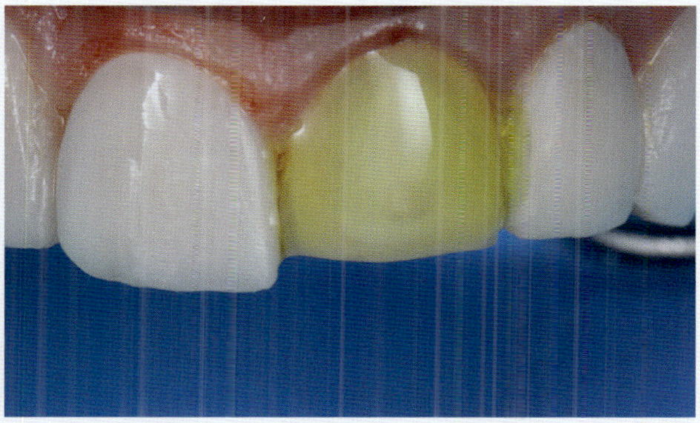

Figure 23

Following building the palatal wall using the silicone index, Unica matrix was placed to complete the frame that should be in accordance with the adjacent teeth as explained above (📷 24, 25).
The dentin shade was applied and mamelons were drawn, leaving a small space in the incisal edge for the translucent material (📷 26).
Si E (Si Enamel) was placed on top in order to give the restoration the translucency and the opalescence properties needed (📷 27).

Left lateral restoration

Always make sure when cutting the mock-up to keep the interproximal references of the adjacent teeth (📷 28-30).

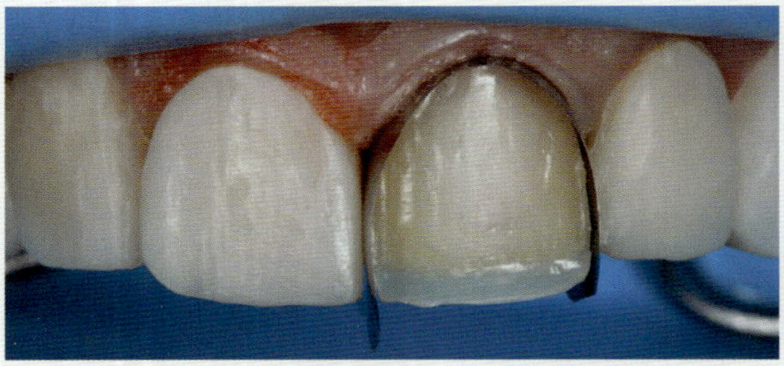
Figure 24

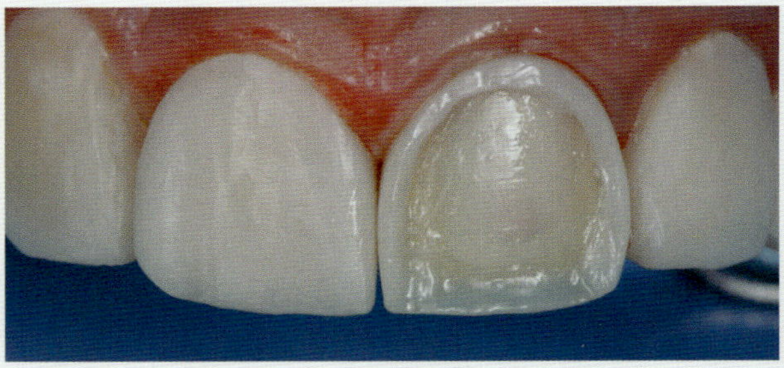
Figure 25

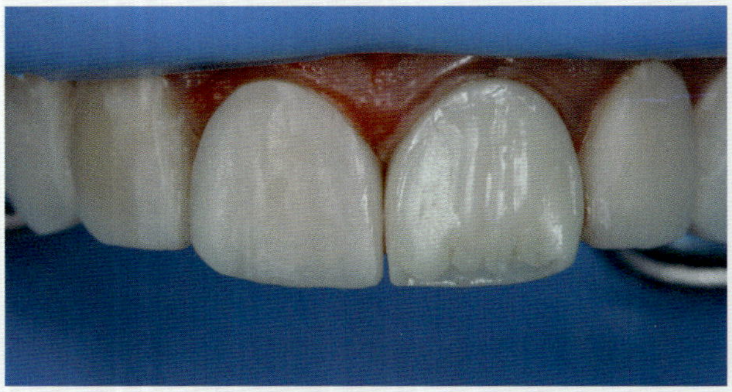
Figure 26

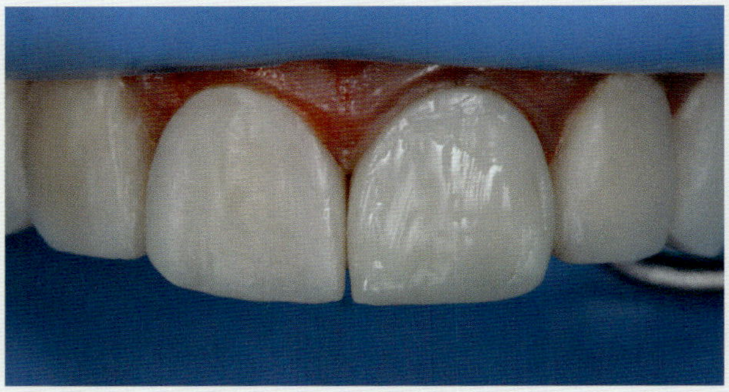
Figure 27

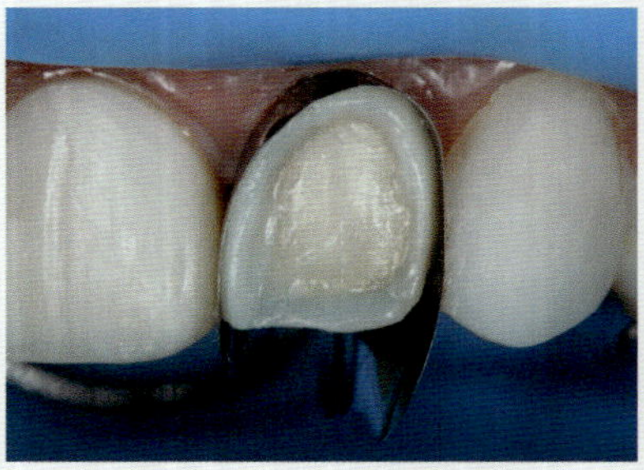
Figure 28

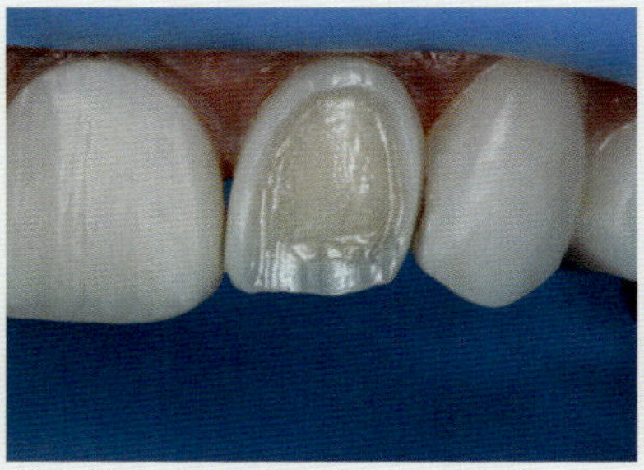
Figure 29

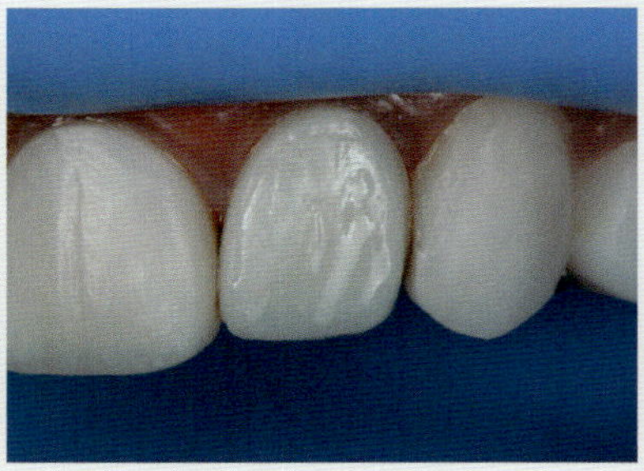
Figure 30

Right lateral restoration

In case of any emergency, we can delay the treatment because the smile is already complete with the mock-up in place on the remaining teeth (31-33).

Right canine restoration

The references to be considered are:

- incisal position: reconstructed using the palatal index (Si E, white dental beauty)
- mesial wall: at the same level than the distal wall of the lateral (Si 0.5, white dental beauty)
- distal wall: at the same level than the mesial wall of the premolar (34-36).

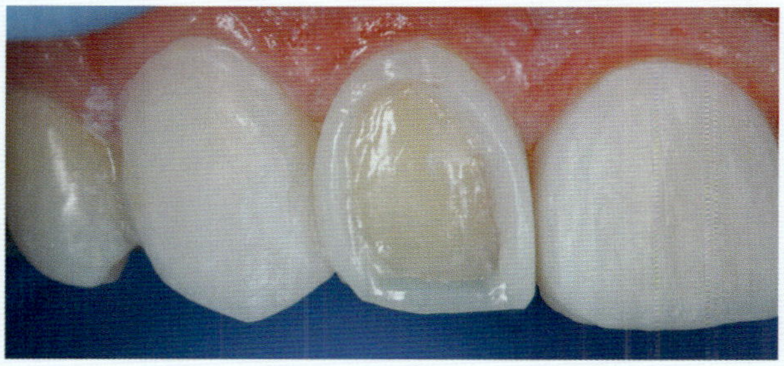

Figure 31

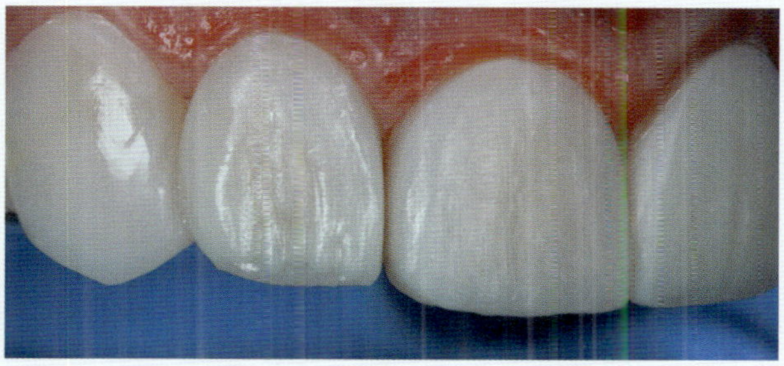

Figure 32

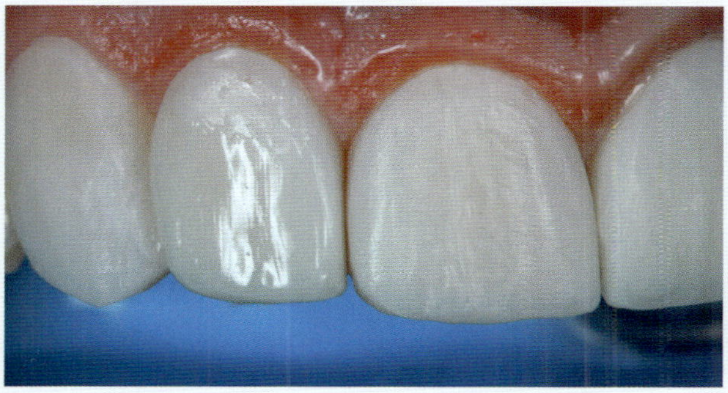

Figure 33

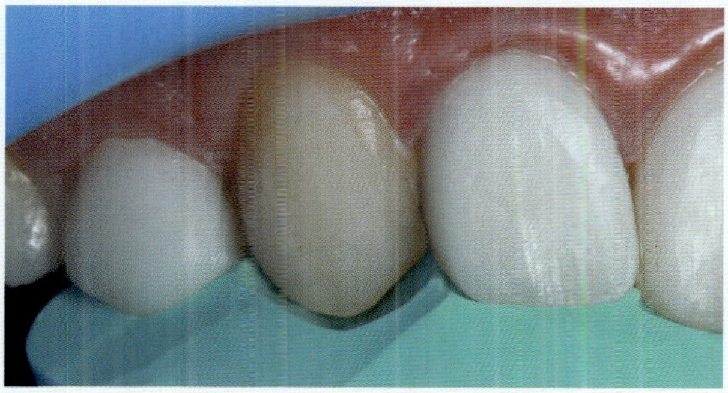

Figure 34

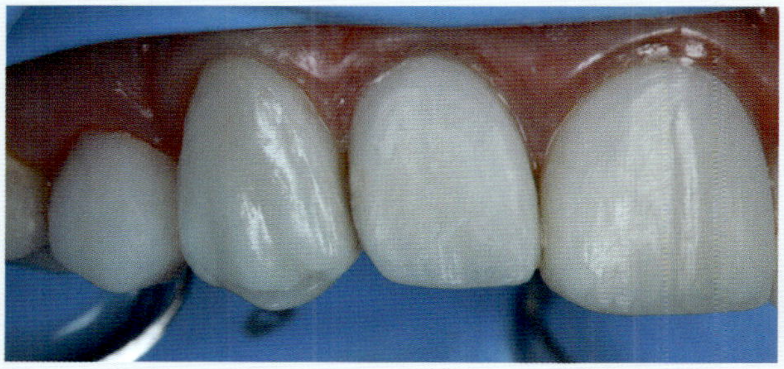

Figure 35

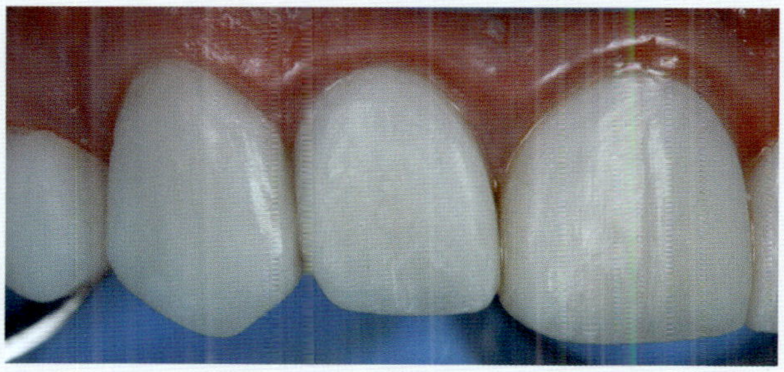

Figure 36

Left canine restoration

After completing all eight restorations, it is well noticed that the final aesthetic outcome is almost achieved. Small details need to be corrected followed by texture and polishing steps (📷 37-39).

Finishing and polishing steps were completed as mentioned in the presented order (📷 40).

Final intraoral picture after polishing with lucida system (📷 41-44).

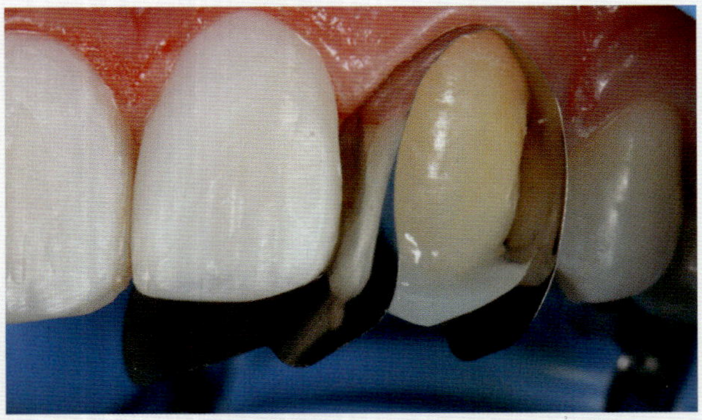

Figure 37

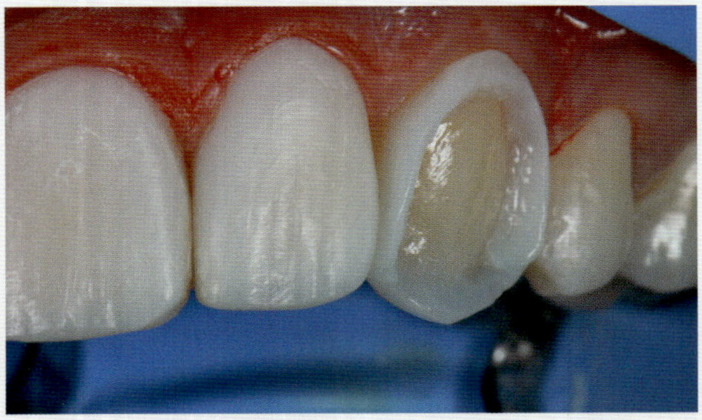

Figure 38

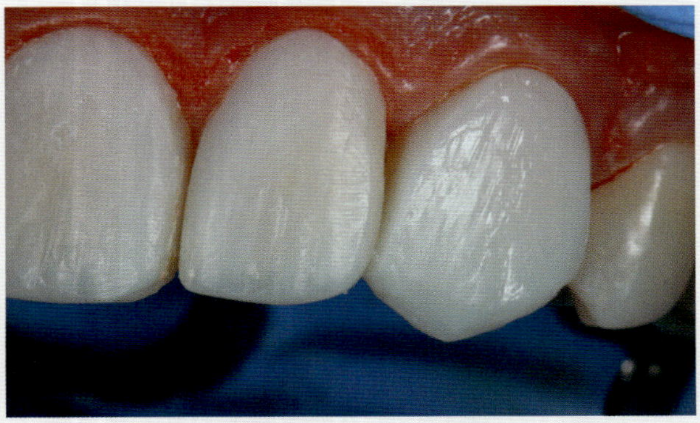

Figure 39

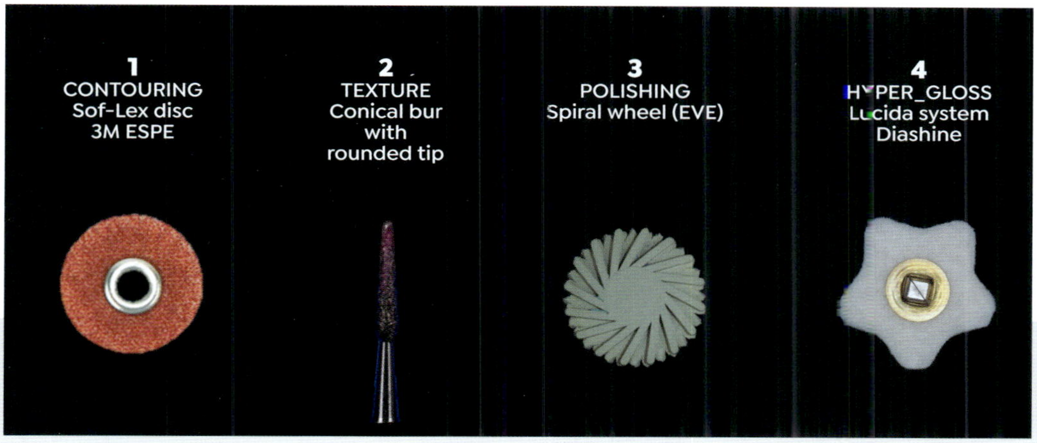

Figure 40

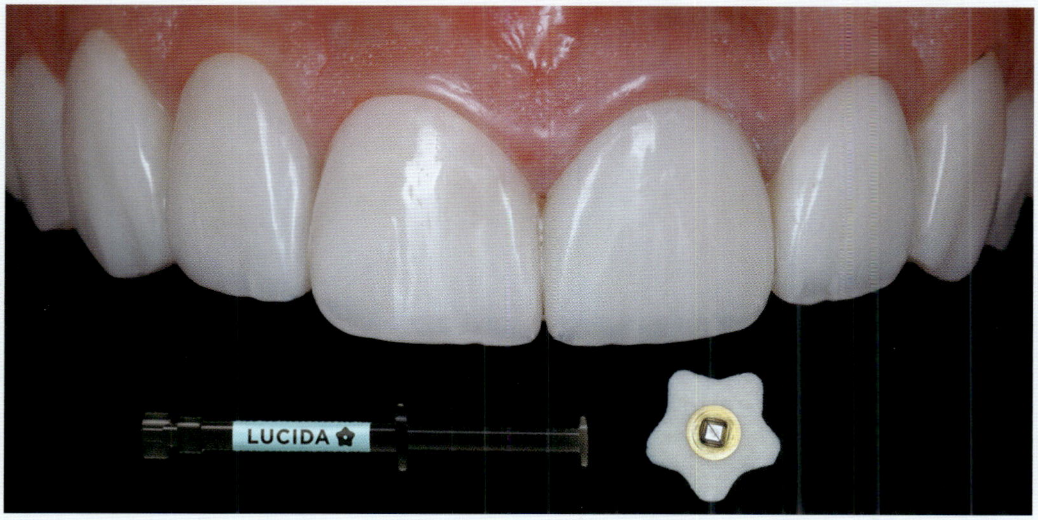

Figure 41

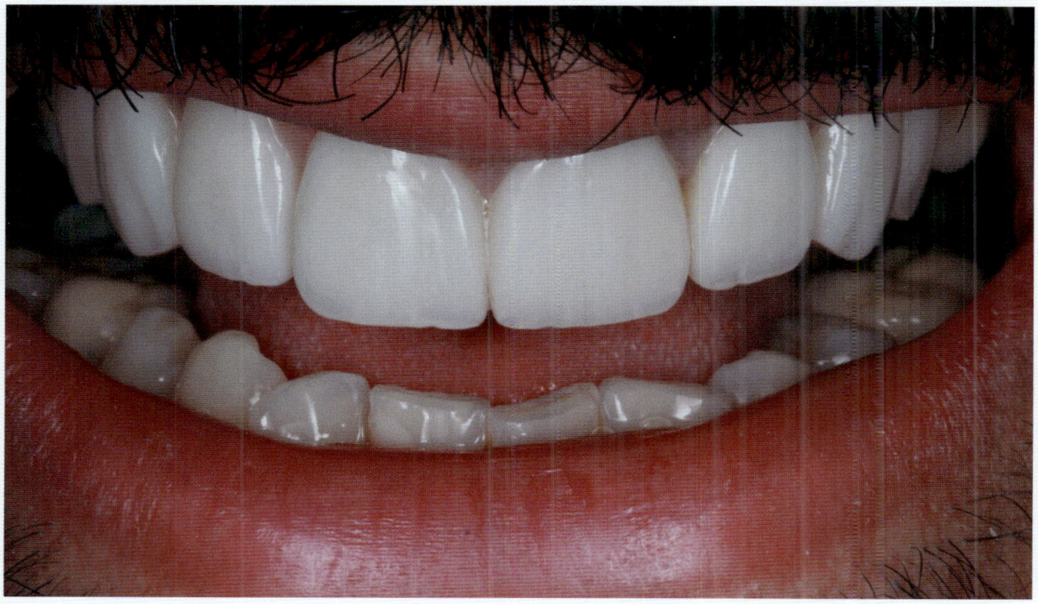

Figure 42

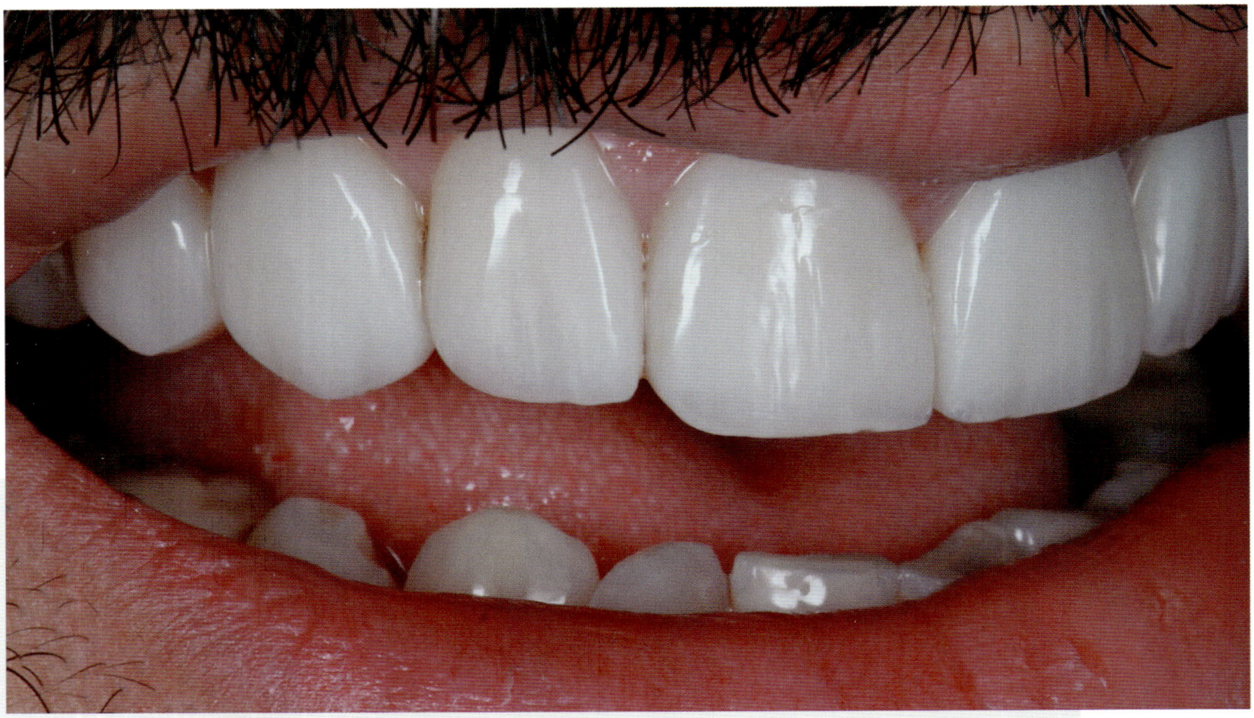

Figure 43

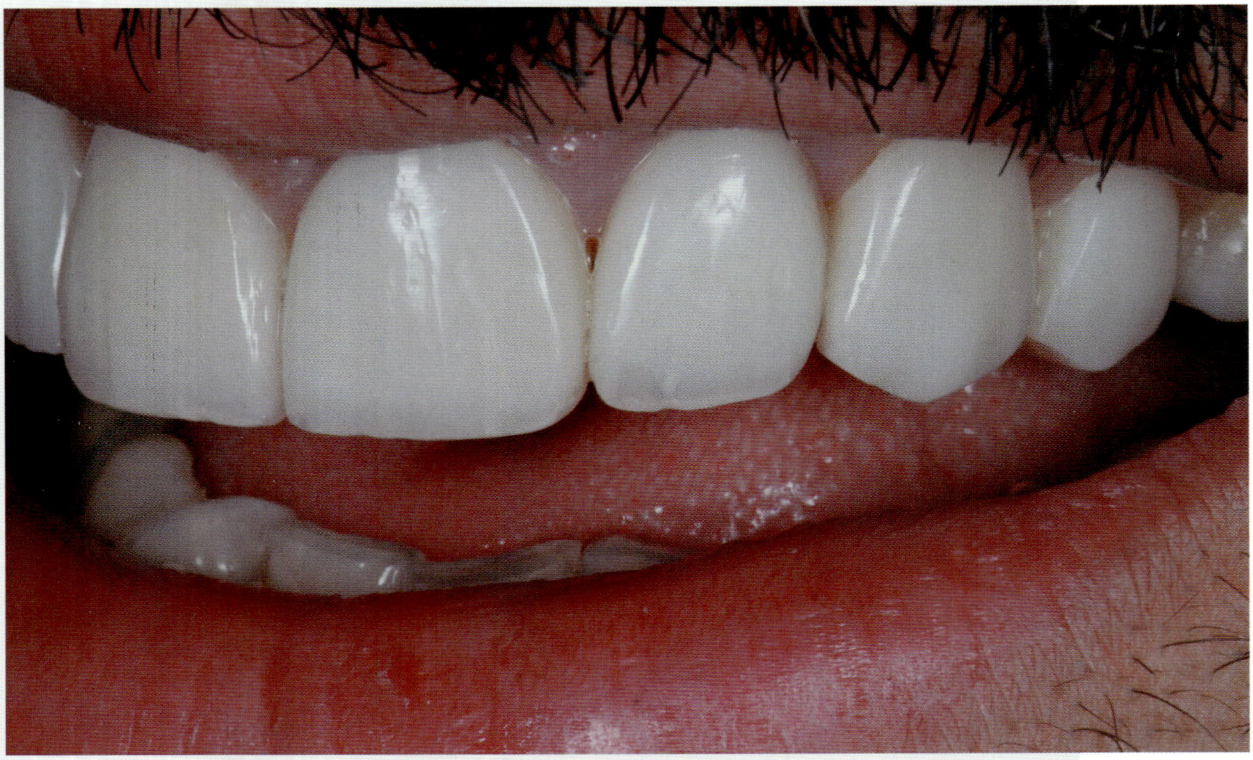

Figure 44

CONCLUSION

The Vestibular Index technique is a simple, reproducible and time saving approach to achieve highly aesthetic direct composite veneers. It allows transforming a complex case into a simple one by only following precisely and easily, a mock-up initially validated by the patient and the dentist. It offers the possibility to finish the treatment in one session or to divide the workflow into two sessions while the patient is still having a complete smile with the provisional restorations in place. It is recommended to use it in medium and complex cases. For simple ones, free hand technique can be enough to achieve the best result.

SUGGESTED READINGS

- Alqarawi FK, Alhumaidan AA, Aldakhili A et al. Intraoral repair of fractured ceramics: a literature review [version 1; peer review: 1 approved]. *F1000Research*. 2022;11:1275.
- Devoto W, Saracinelli M, Manauta J. Composite in everyday practice: how to choose the right material and simplify application techniques in the anterior teeth. *Eur J Esthet Dent*. 2010;5:102-124.
- Dietschi D. Optimizing smile composition and esthetics with resin composites and other conservative esthetic procedures. *Eur J Esthet Dent*. 2008;3(1):14-29.
- Dietschi D, Shahidi C, Krejci I. Clinical performance of direct anterior composite restorations: a systematic literature review and critical appraisal. *Int J Esthet Dent*. 2019;14:252-270.
- Manauta J, Salat A. *Layers, An atlas of composite resin stratification*. Quintessence Publishing, 2012.
- Manauta J, Salat A, Devoto W, Putignano A. *Layers 2. Direct Composites: The Styleitaliano Clinical Secrets*. Quintessence Publishing, 2022.
- Paolone G, Orsini G, Manauta J et al. Composite shade guides and color matching. *Int J Esthet Dent*. 2014;9(2):164-182.

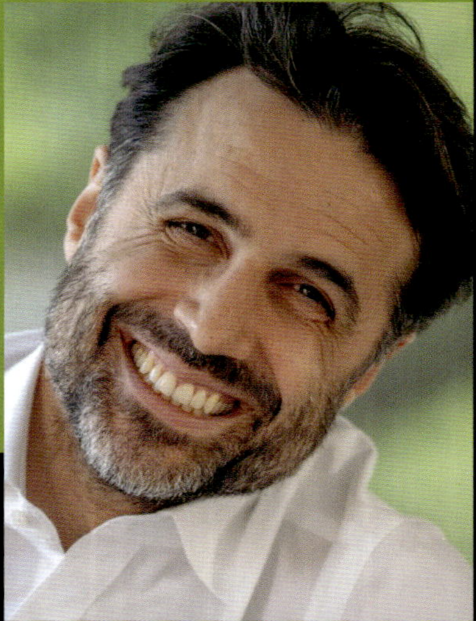

GIUSEPPE CHIODERA

Italy

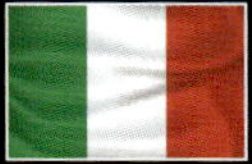

Giuseppe Chiodera graduated in dentistry from the University of Brescia. In 2004 he was the winner of a scholarship at King's College London University.
He is an honorary member of the StyleItaliano group.
Author and co-author of several publications in national and international journals, he is a speaker at national and international conferences.
He practices in a private practice, devoting himself mainly to conservative and aesthetic dentistry.

FRAMING A SMILE

In recent years we have witnessed a steady growth in aesthetic demands made by patients.
They are accompanied by expectations that need to find concrete, but also realistic, answers. Determining a frame and defining the limits of the smile are fundamental actions to allow the technician to design a new one or to allow us to build the new aesthetic freehand. Within this frame will be our manual dexterity, aesthetic sensitivity, empathy toward the patient, passion for details and for our work.

DISCUSSION AND CLINICAL CASES

Increasingly, thanks to new materials, tools, techniques, and the widespread influence of social media, patients are asking to transform their smiles. They do not just desire the care of a single tooth, but aim to improve the overall appearance of their smile (📷 1, 2). To meet this need, we need a framework that demarcates the space within which we can either reconstruct directly at the chairside or have the laboratory design the reconstruction. This space essentially consists of three parts:

- gingival parabolas
- occlusal arch
- midline.

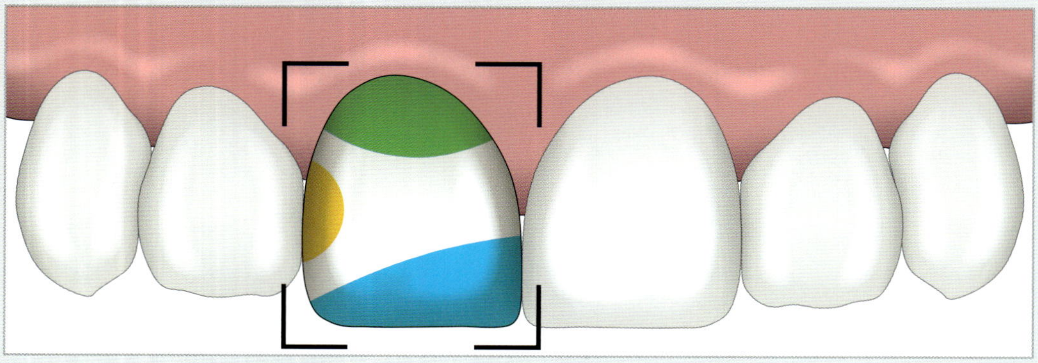

Figure 1

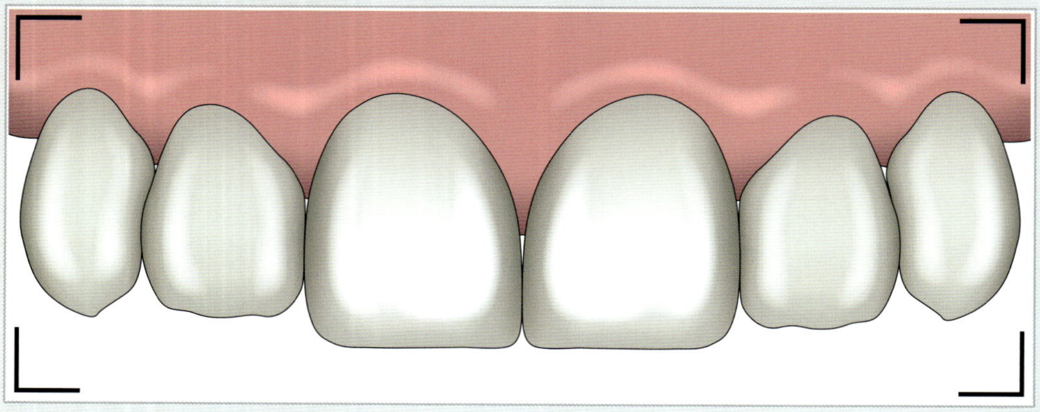

Figure 2

At the materials level, when we manage a smile in its entirety, we use dedicated composites with high opacity and mimetic ability to minimize the use of different masses. Layering many masses in small restorations can lead to the inclusion of bubbles in the restoration, visible during the polishing phase (3). Therefore, it is preferable to work on large restorations with fewer masses.

Compared to the ideal smile, the patient may perceive the transition lines as discordant and aesthetically unappealing; therefore, there should be no teeth with straight and other curved transition lines, as this would be unpleasant (4, 5). Even an ordinary observer will easily notice inadequately open embrasures (6), as well as perceive the oblique midline between the two centrals as something disharmonious (7).

A factor easily perceived by patients as unpleasant is when the parabolas are on different levels, especially in patients who smile showing gingival margins (8).

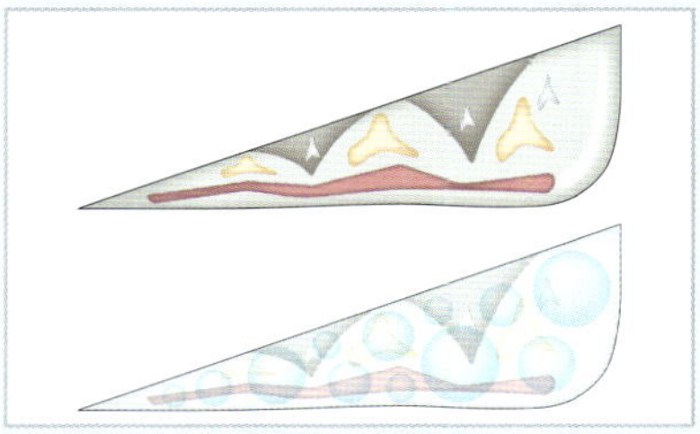

Figure 3

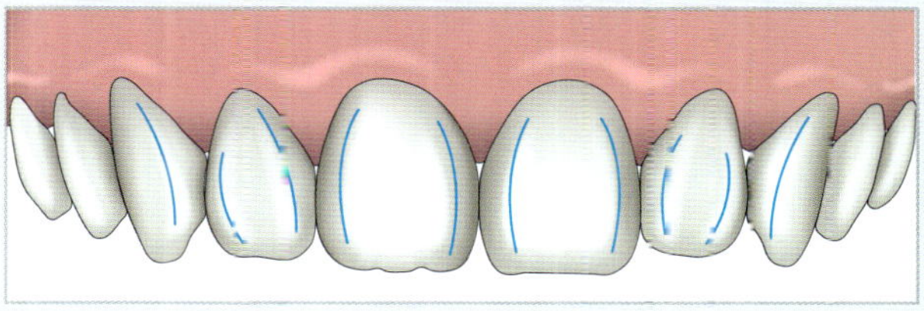

Figure 4

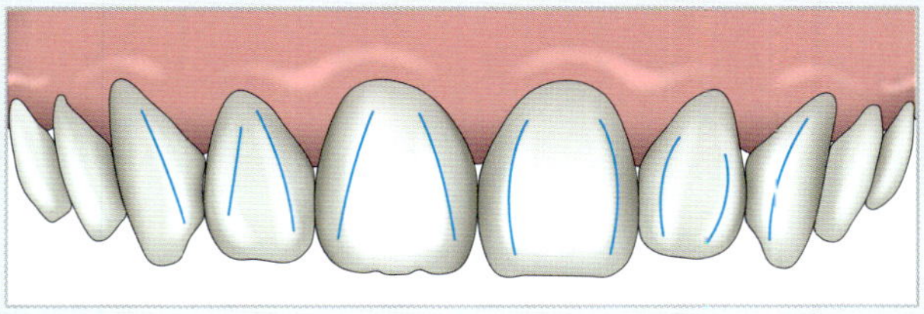

Figure 5

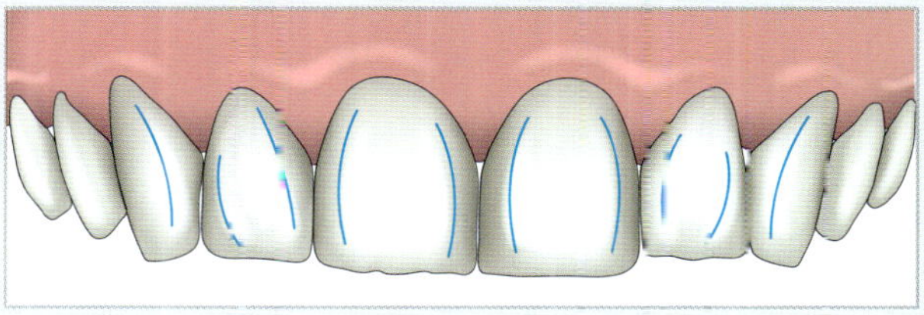

Figure 6

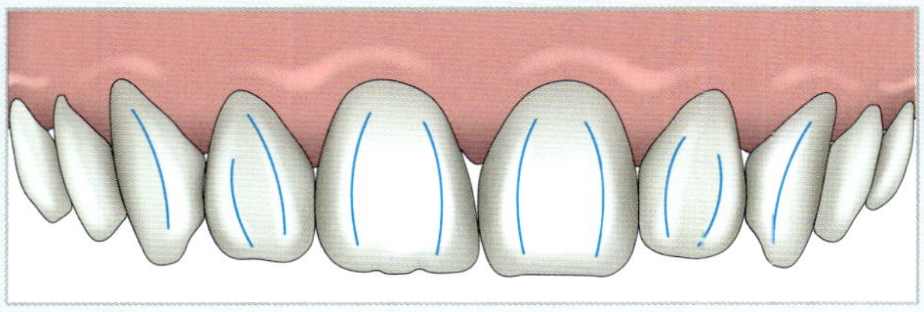

Figure 7

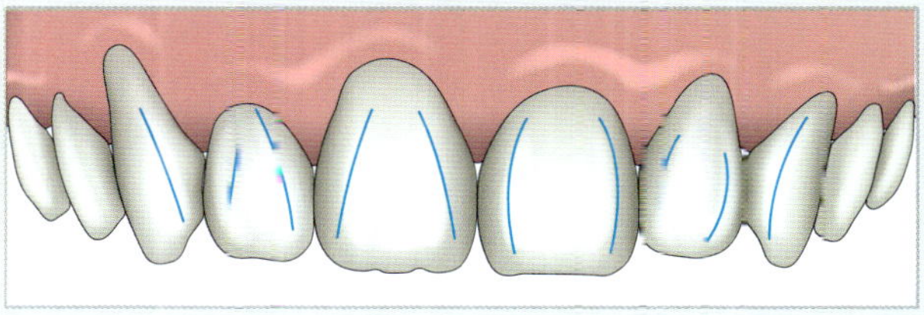

Figure 8

When a patient seeks aesthetic improvement, we must anticipate what he will notice at the end of treatment, not just what he requires at the beginning. His or her ability to perceive aesthetic details will be increasing, and if the restorations are composite, we can make changes during the ongoing work. It is crucial to plan from the beginning the correct position of the parabolas and make the arch of the smile homogeneous from an occlusal view **(📷 9)**. Sometimes teeth will be external to the ideal arch **(📷 10)**, other times internal **(📷 11)**. In addition, a laboratory step is sometimes necessary to manage the position of the parabolas as best as possible. In **Figure 12**, the procedure of removing

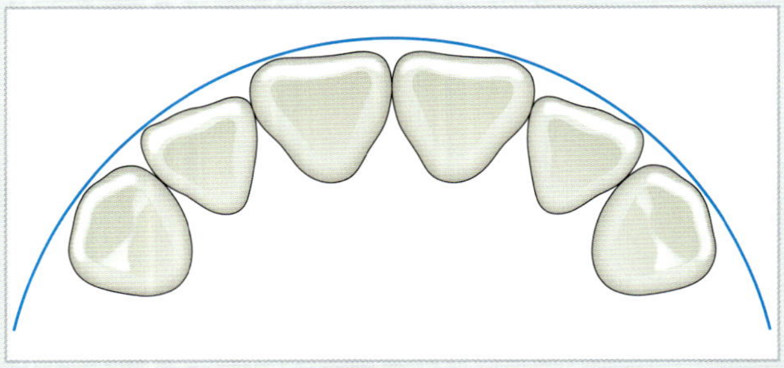

Figure 9

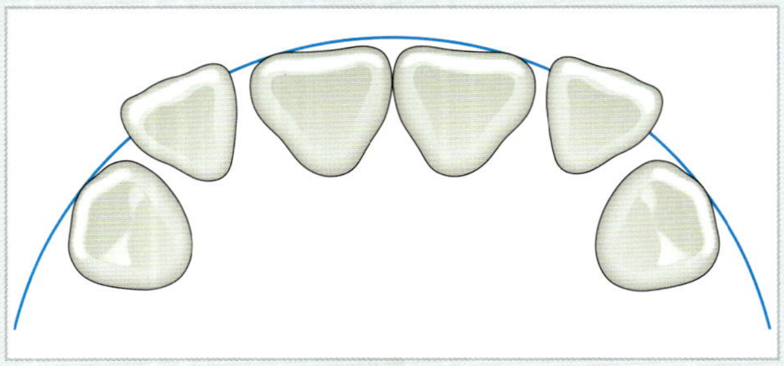

Figure 10

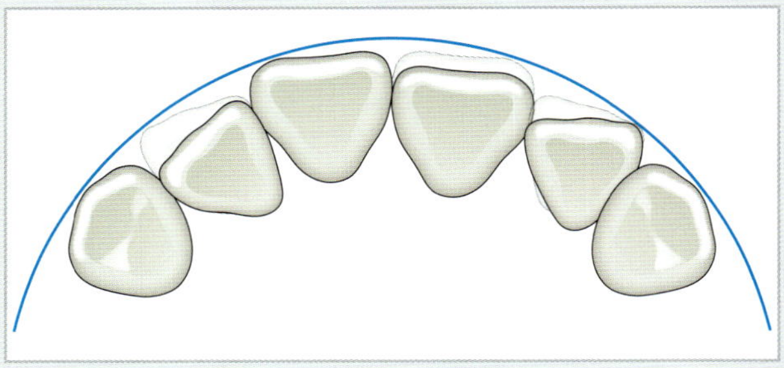

Figure 11

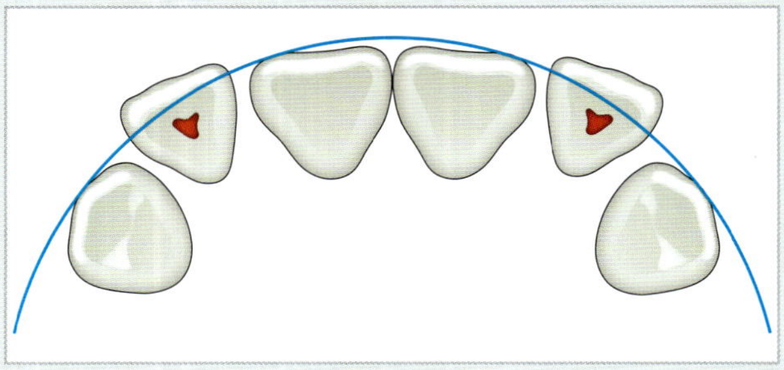

Figure 12

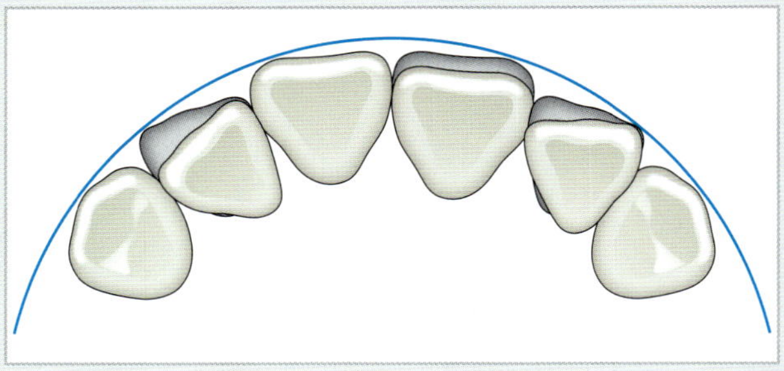

Figure 13

a portion of enamel by targeted ameloplasty to realign the teeth is shown. It is useful to make this cut before requesting the new smile design from the laboratory, whether proceeding analogically with a wax-up or using digital tools.

In **Figure 13**, on the other hand, composite additions are made to achieve a correct arch. In the context of Class V restoration, the use of the LM-Gengiva instrument allows significant relocation of the gingival parabola. In many circumstances, we can move the gingiva to a more cervical position without the need for gingivectomy or surgery (**14**).

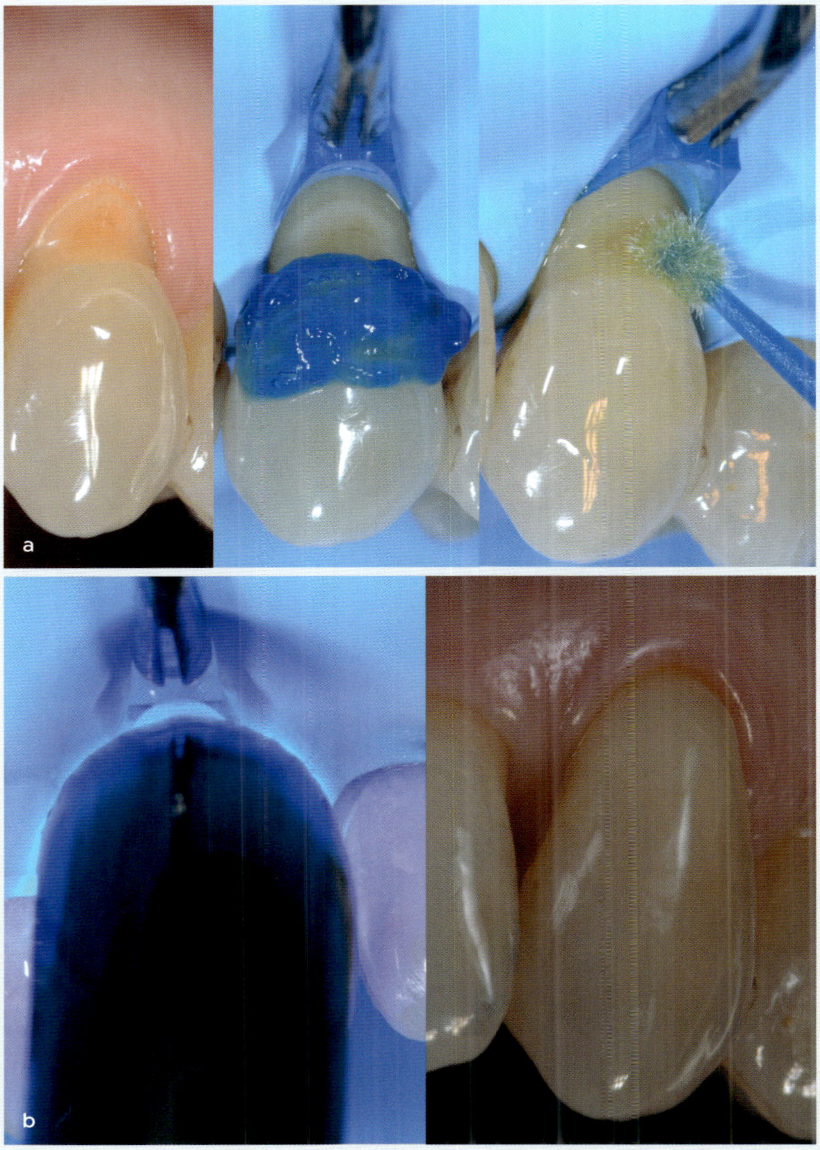

Figure 14

Clinical case 1

In the case of **Figure 15**, we performed direct freehand composite veneers on teeth 12 and 22 without resorting to surgery. As these were two single teeth interspersed with healthy teeth, direct reconstruction was possible.

In **Figure 16**, the parabolas are corrected in height, and we will have to make multiple Class V restorations that will be part of the direct composite veneers on all teeth except the ceramic of 2.2. Thus, we will rebuild the harmony of the smile. With Class V and LM-Gengiva restorations, we can redesign the shape of the parabolas to make them more harmonious with the new crown on 1.2 **(📷 17)**.

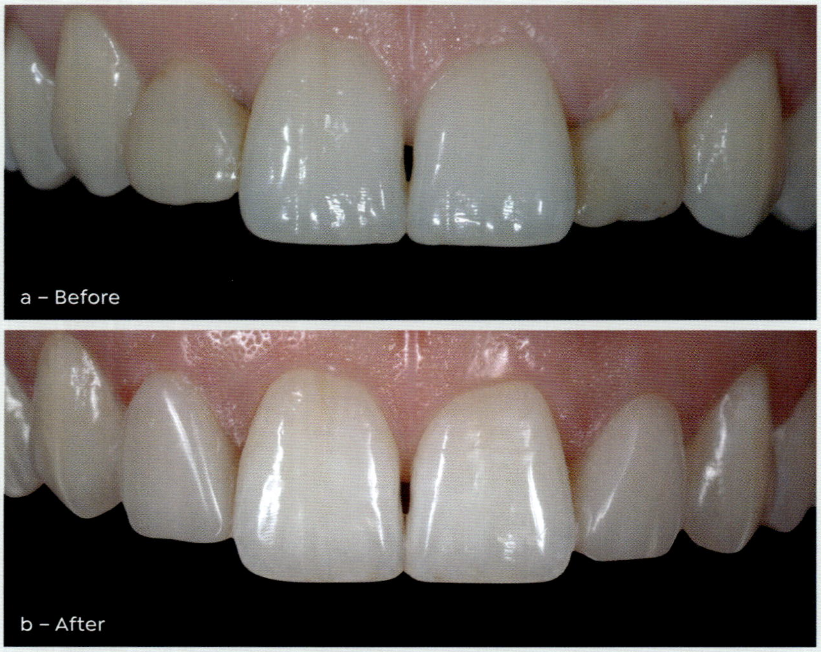

Figure 15

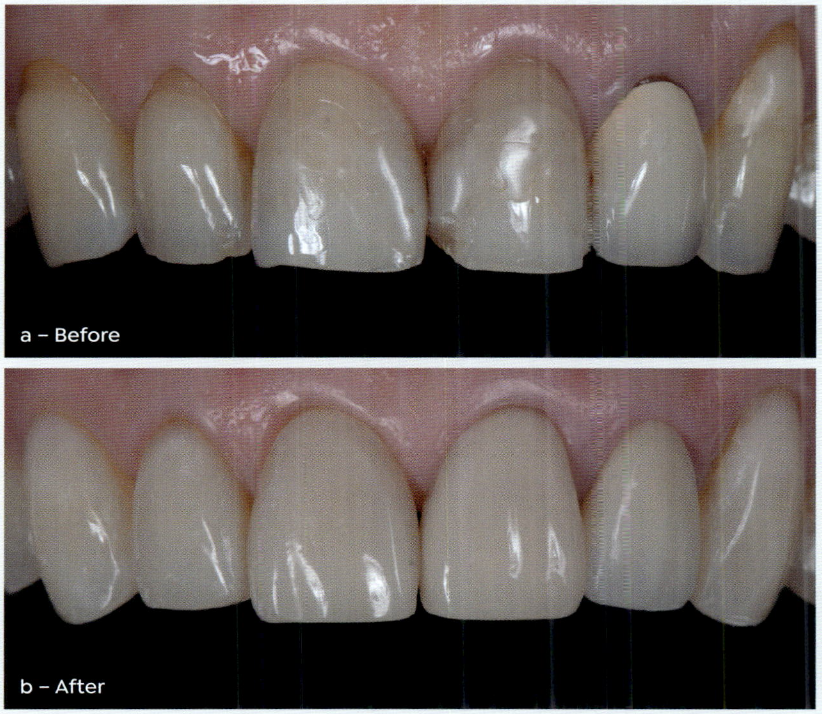

Figure 16

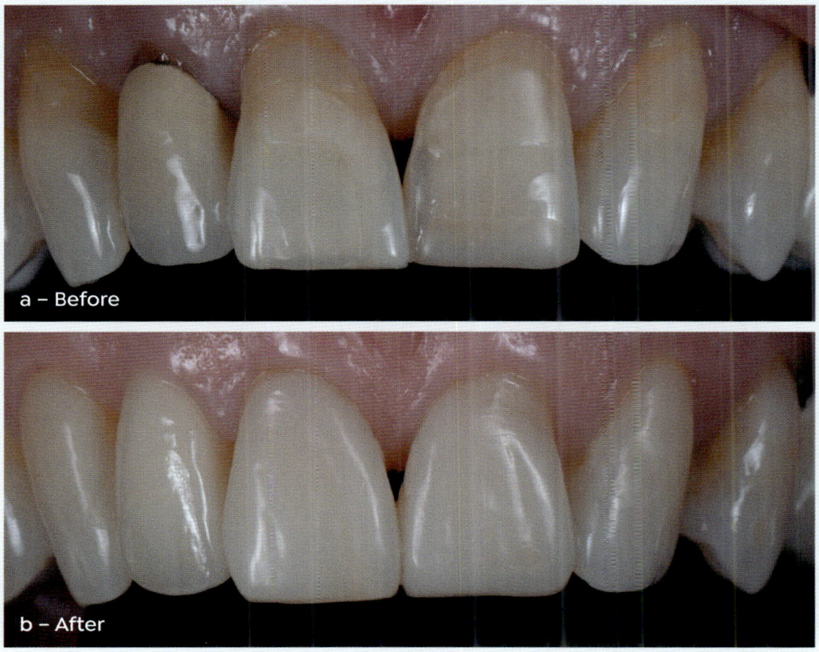

Figure 17

Clinical case 2

In the case of multiple remakes of Class V restorations in a patient in whom we are going to prosthesize posterior sections 1 and 2, it was proposed to realign the anterior teeth in composite. Once again, we were able to harmonize the composite parabolas on the upper four central teeth (18-24).

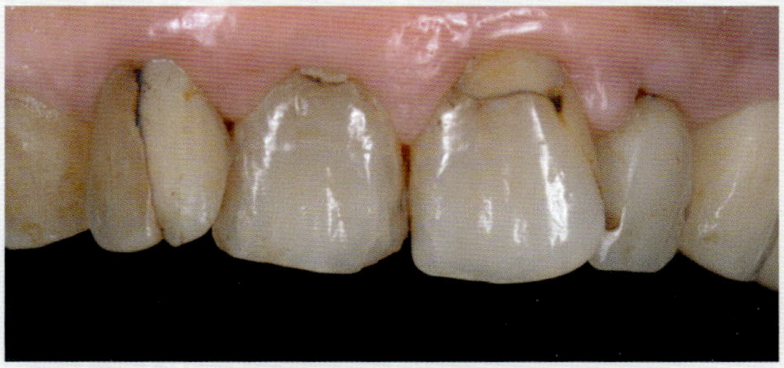

Figure 18

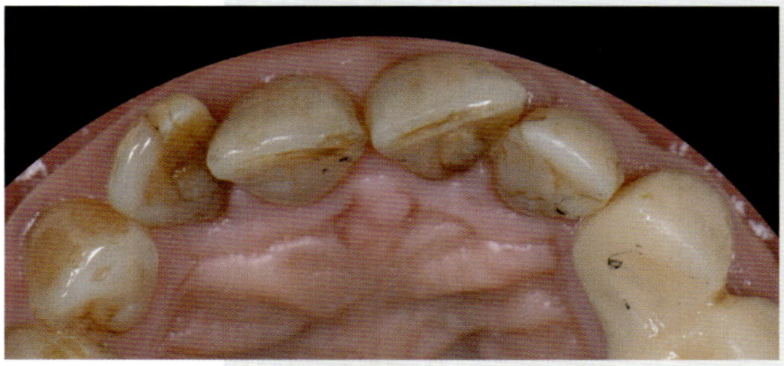

Figure 19 Initial case image in occlusal view, where the misalignment of the teeth can be better assessed.

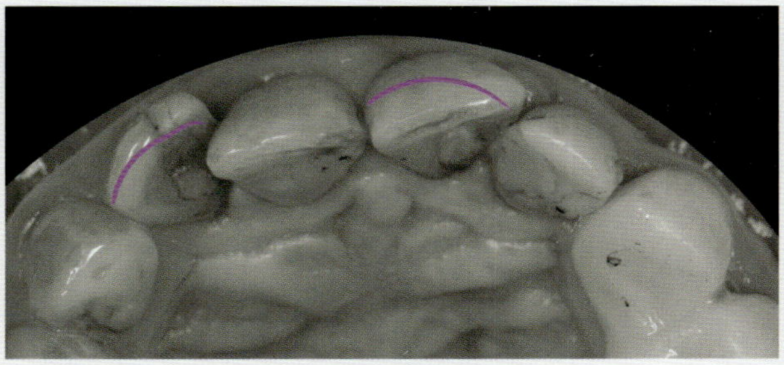

Figure 20 Highlighted in pink are the points where we should go for vestibular changes in the teeth to harmonize the smile.

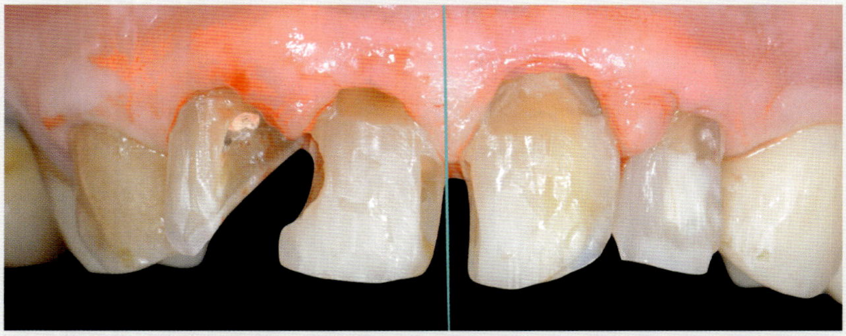

Figure 21 Removal of old composites and ameloplasties performed with copious irrigation without anesthesia to minimize the risk of postoperative sensitivity and pulpal exposure. After preparations, we verify that the turquoise midline is positioned between the two central incisors; if not, we will evaluate further ameloplasty procedures on 11 mesial. Whether reconstructing teeth freehand or with a lab-provided guide, it is critical to have adequate spaces.

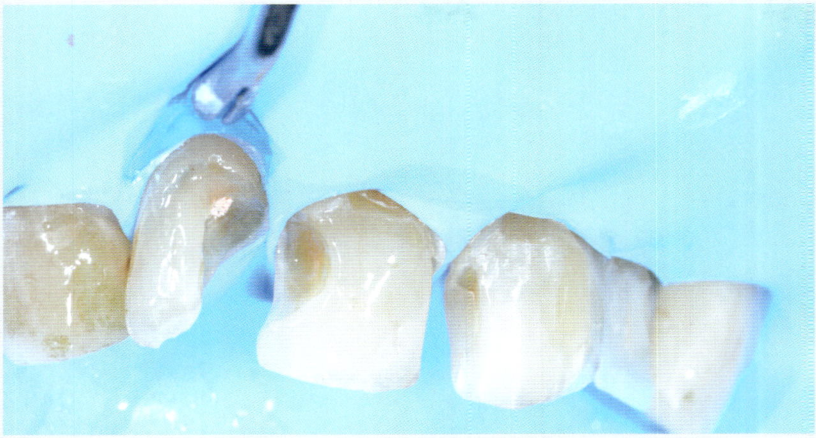

Figure 22 Detail of collar reconstruction with LM-Gengiva.

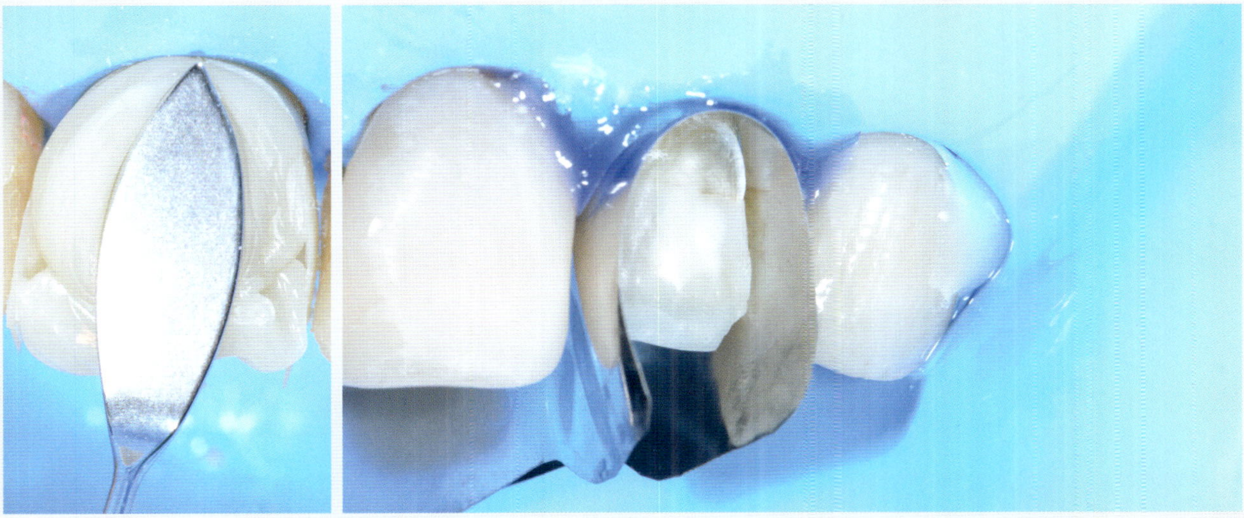

Figure 23 In this case, the Unica matrix of Polycentia, the composite veneer modeled with Solo Anterior LM, is used to apically relocate the parabola of 2.2.

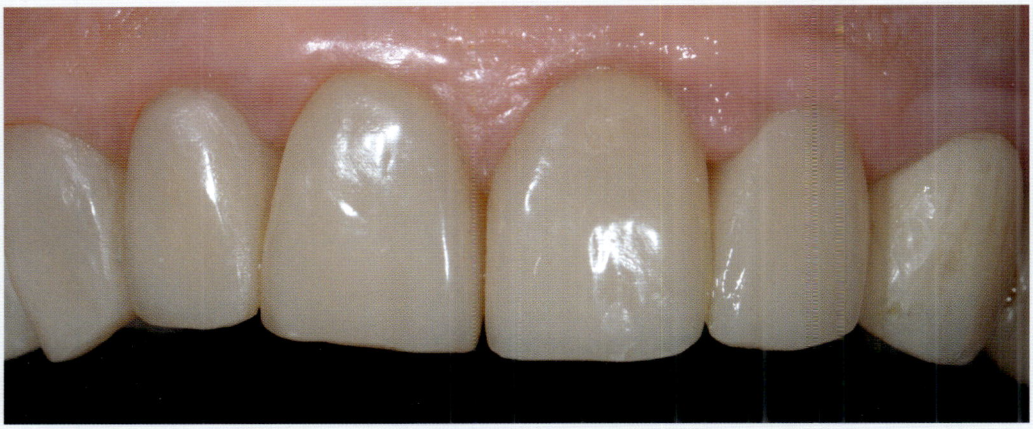

Figure 24

Clinical case 3

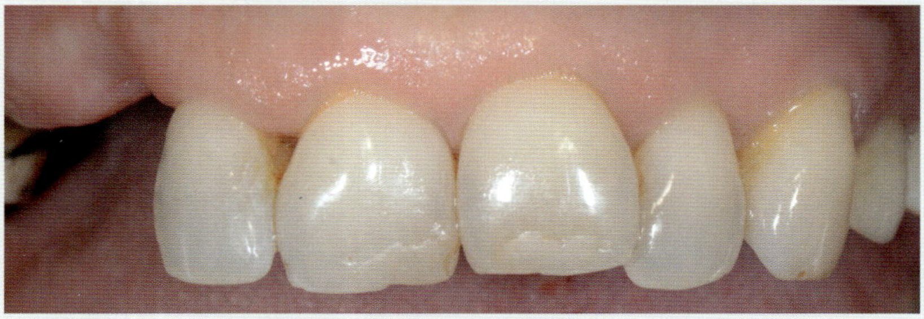

Figure 25 Initial case image.

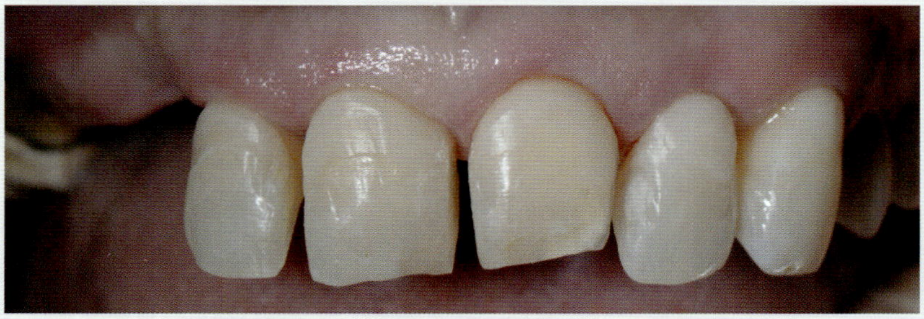

Figure 26 The frame is ready, we performed ameloplasty on 21 because vestibularized, repositioned the misaligned collars, without the dam. Looking at the patient's face, we verified that the correct median passes over the mesial wall of tooth 11.

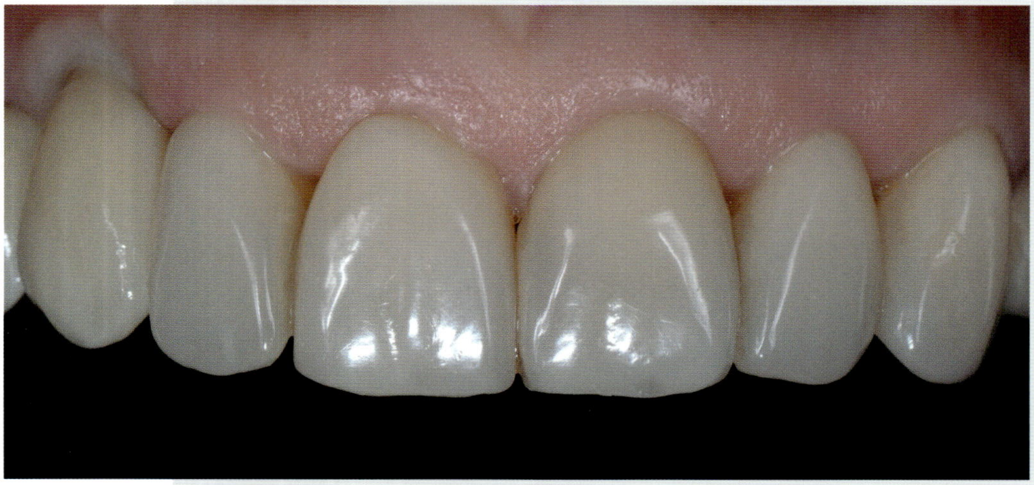

Figure 27 We can then proceed to direct veneers on all teeth, guided by the lab or freehand; the more teeth, the more support from the lab will be helpful.

In the diagram in **Figure 28** we observe how the laboratory, with a diagnostic wax-up D, can change the position of the parabolas, showing us with the wax-up where they should be placed. The problem might arise once this information is transferred and printed on the patient, as shown in the yellow portion of figure D. Sometimes this is feasible, sometimes not, and surgery may be necessary. Either way, this can generate stress for us and the patient.

In the diagram in **Figure 29**, the procedure becomes more streamlined if we provide the technician with the cervical position. If we have already repositioned the parabolas in a preliminary appointment, this approach will allow the diagnostic wax-up information to be transferred, printed, and injected always under dam.

We see this approach in clinical cases 4 and 5.

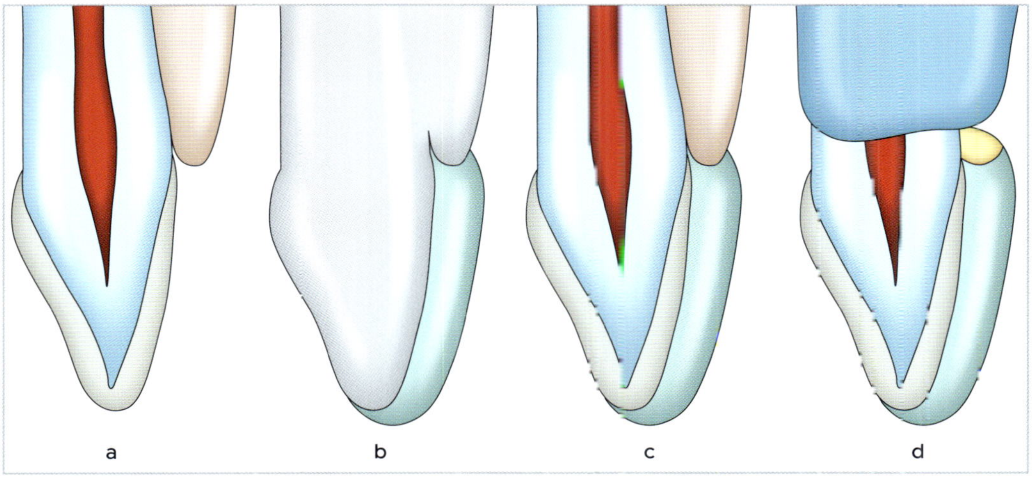

Figure 28

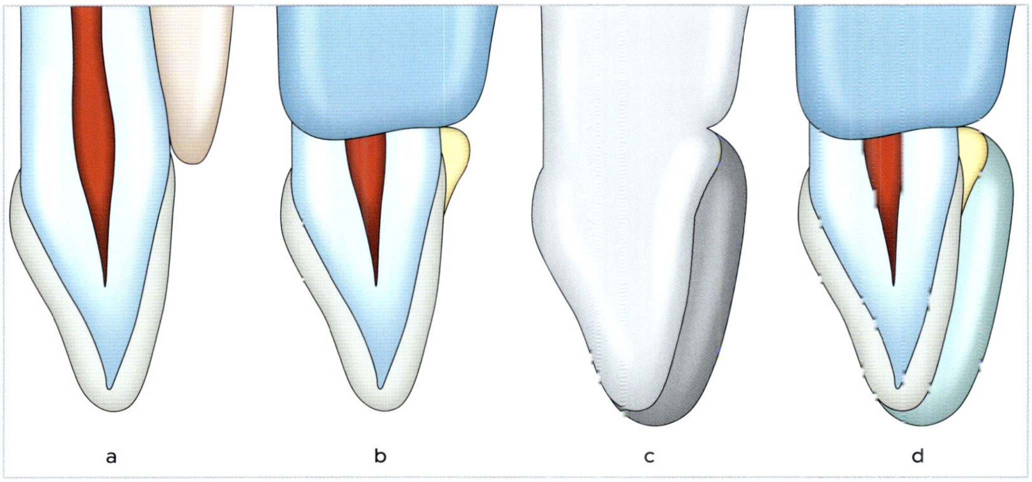

Figure 29

Clinical case 4

Analog wax-up

The patient requires smile improvement and presents with a deep bite **(📷 30)** and severe misalignment of lateral incisors with old restorations **(📷 31, 32)**.

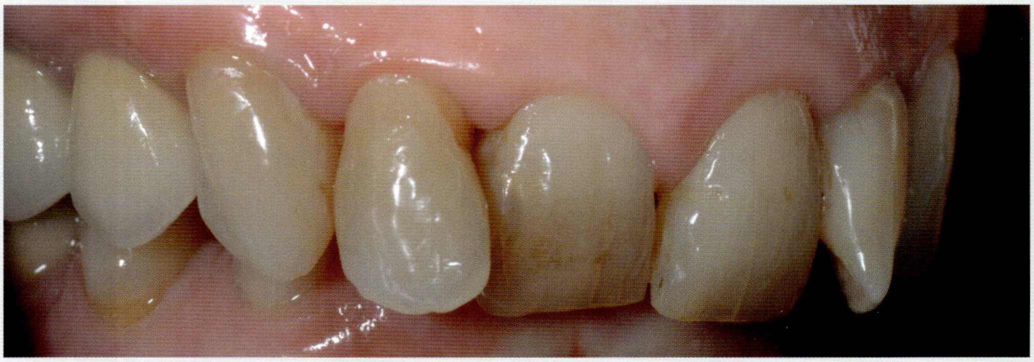

Figure 30

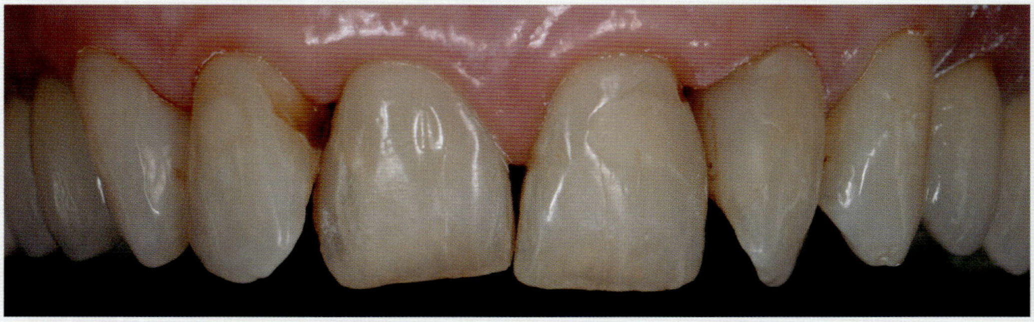

Figure 31

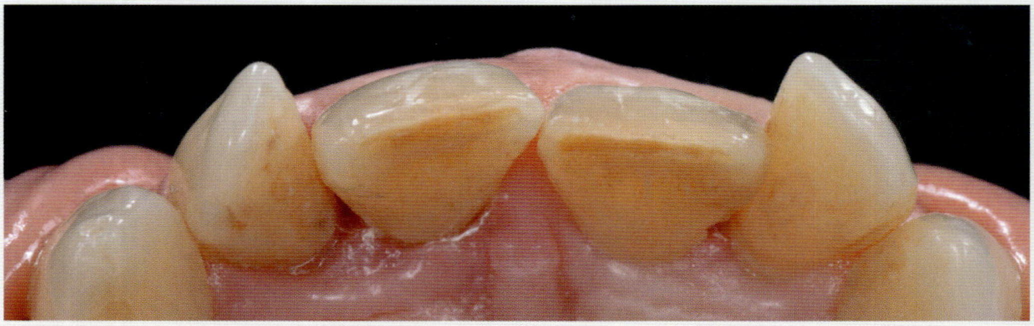

Figure 32

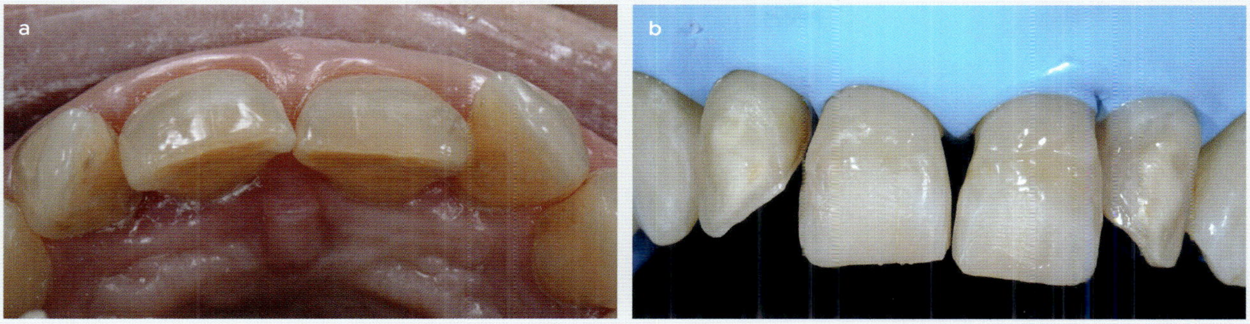

Figure 33 An ameloplasty is performed on the lateral incisors without anesthesia, and the collars are realigned to provide a clear reference for the technician on the cervical position for waxing up the teeth and facilitate field isolation.

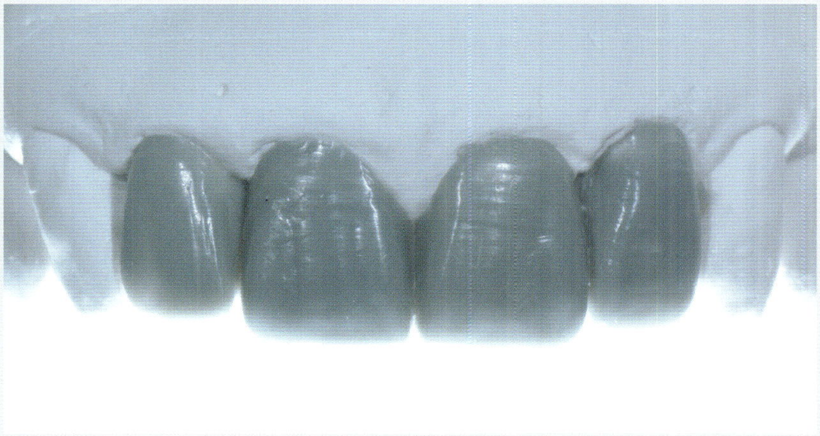

Figure 34 The dental technician can design the wax-up of the four central incisors from the cervical position of the previously reconstructed collars.

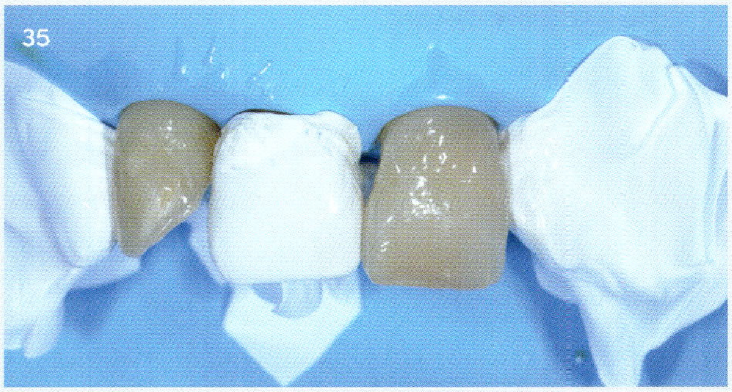

Figures 35-37 It is possible for the dentist to inject flow composite through holes in the incisal portion of the transparent template using the injection molding technique, transferring the information from the diagnostic wax-up onto the teeth (📷 35). The technique involves molding alternating teeth, not all at once. We start by molding 12 21, protecting the neighboring teeth with Teflon, and then molding 11 22, again protecting the neighboring teeth and restorations with Teflon (📷 36, 37).

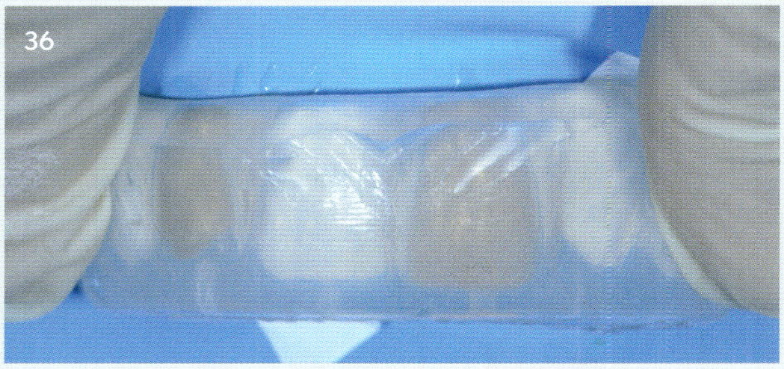

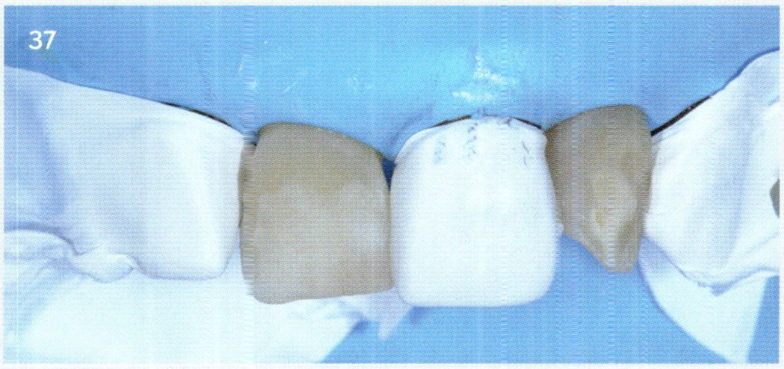

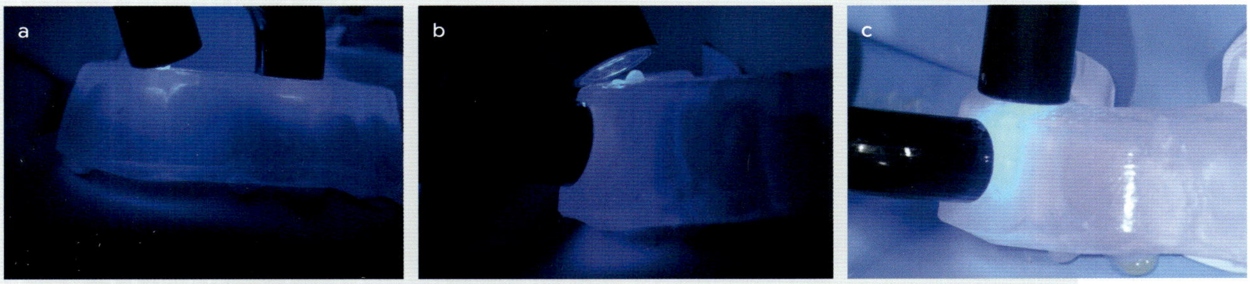

Figure 38 Two-lamp curing is always recommended, either in the incisal region through the access holes (a), or with cross projections of the light beams from the buccal and incisal, as shown in pictures (b) and (c).

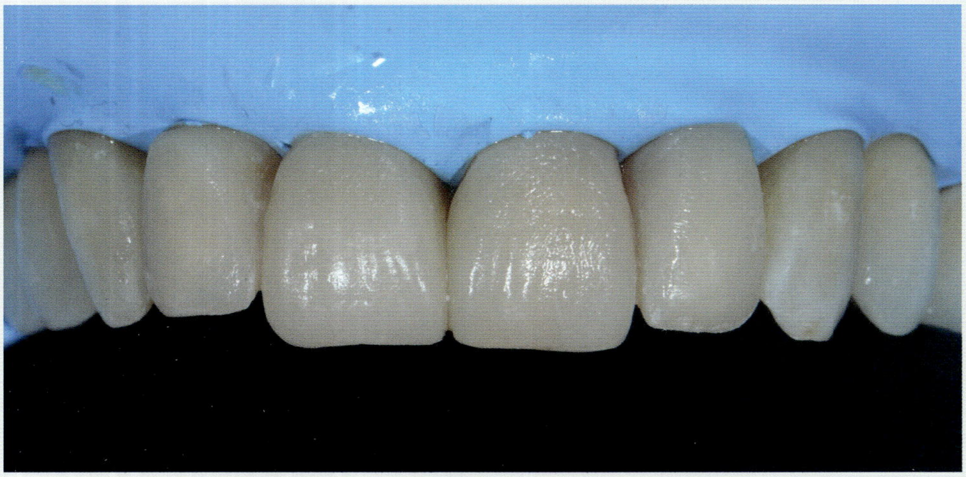

Figure 39 Completed restorations under dam.

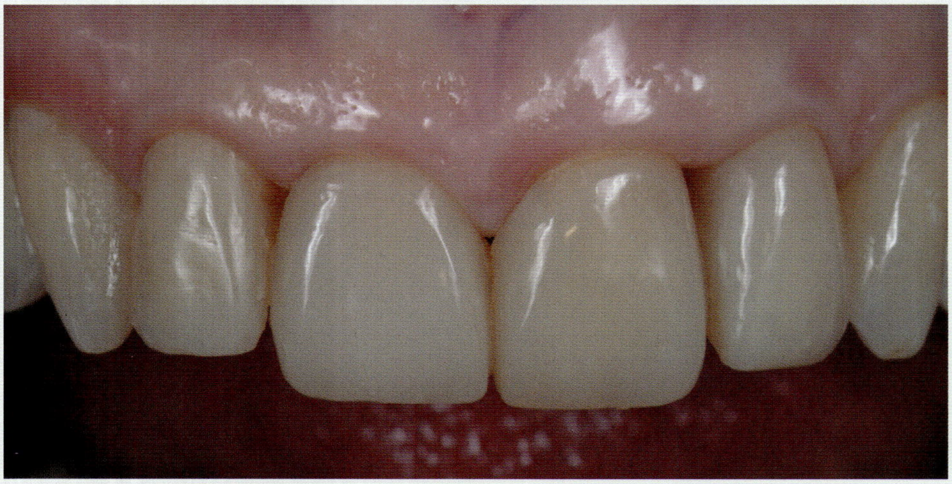

Figure 40 Restorations polished with LUCIDA DiaShine®.

Clinical case 5
Digital wax-up

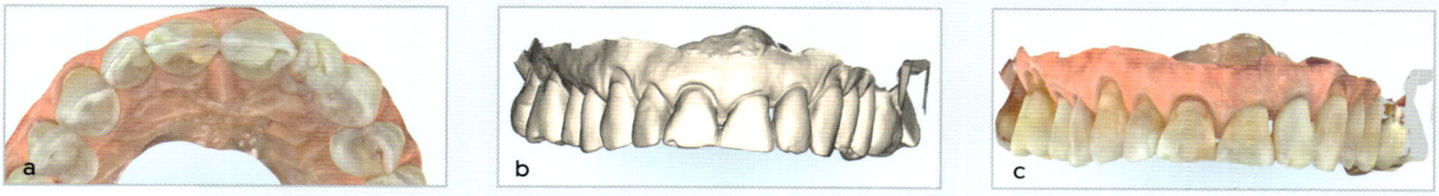

Figure 41 Preliminary scan at the start of treatment with the iTeroTM intraoral scanner.

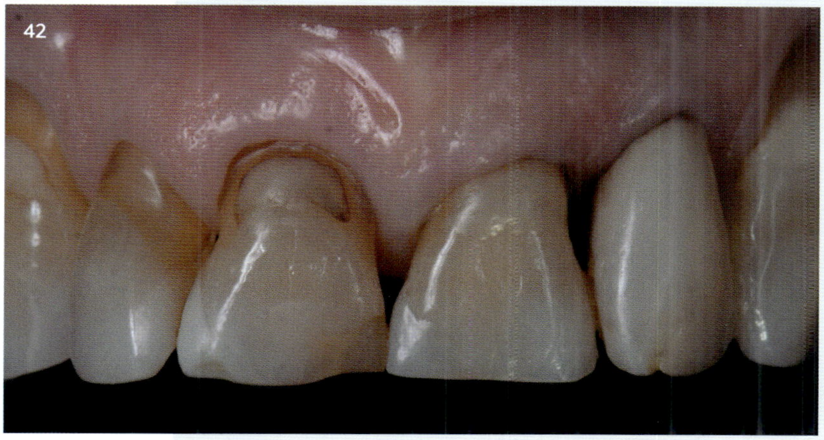

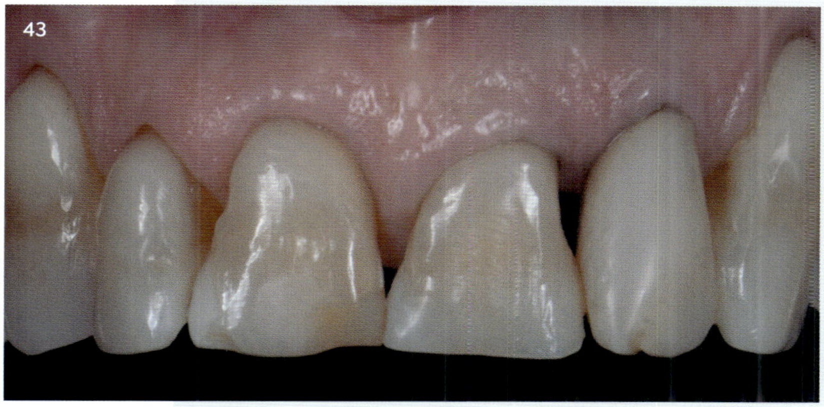

Figures 42, 43 The first crucial step is to construct the frame, removing the old restorations to replace them with the new ones. At the same time, the composite collars are repositioned.

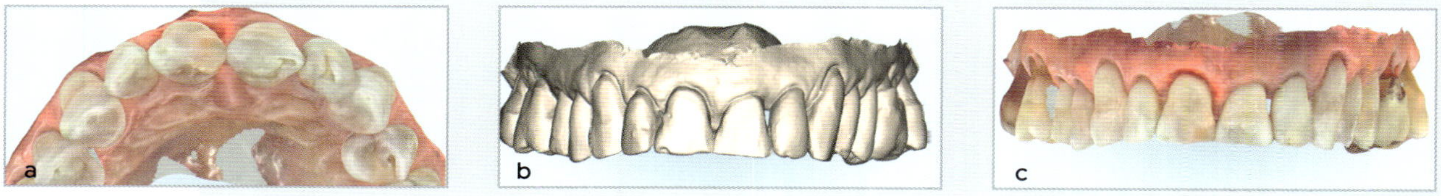

Figure 44 Completed scan at the end of the first treatment step.

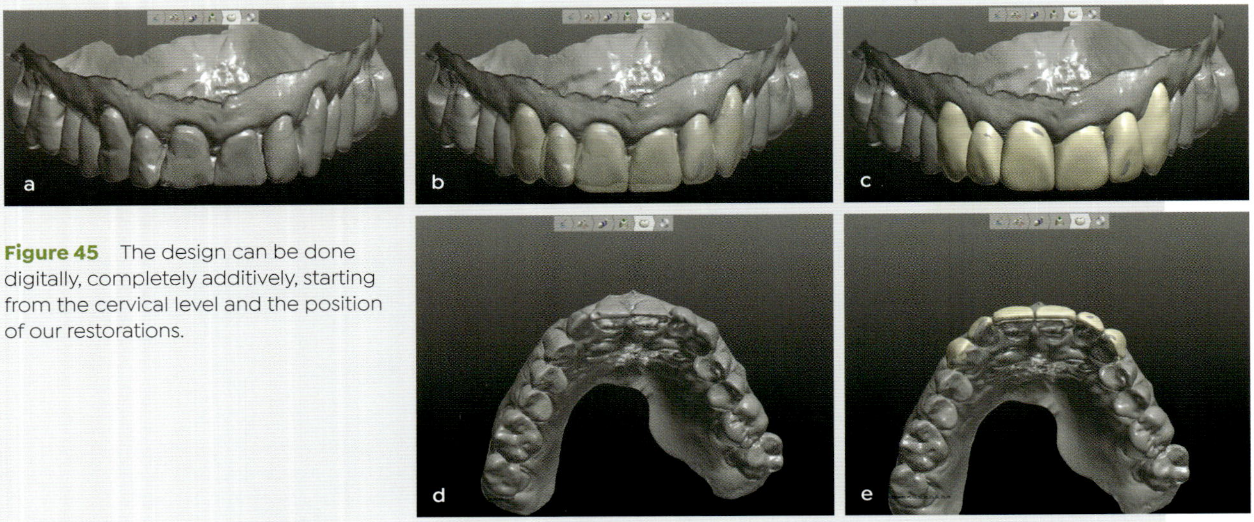

Figure 45 The design can be done digitally, completely additively, starting from the cervical level and the position of our restorations.

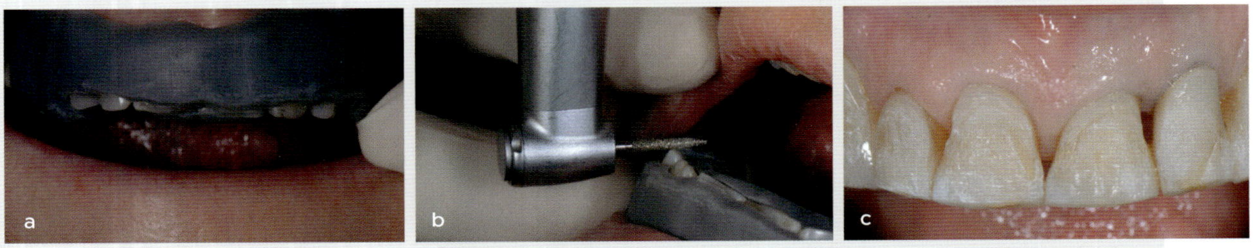

Figure 46 It is up to us, our expertise and the strategy planned with the patient, to decide whether to proceed with direct, semi-direct or innovative techniques such as Styloso.

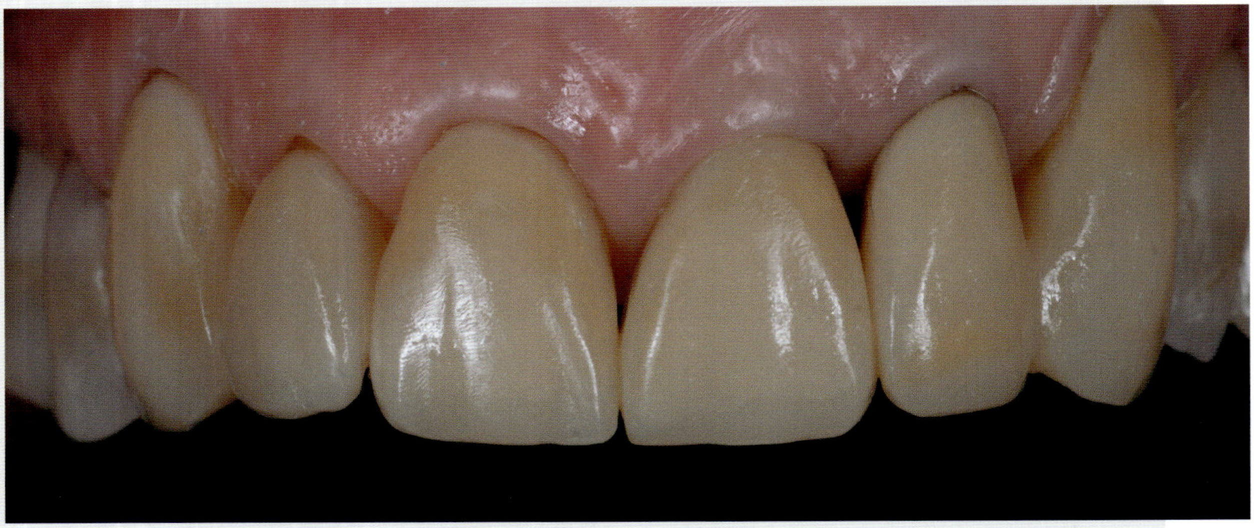

Figure 47 Image of completed restorations.

CONCLUSION

However we decide to rehabilitate a patient in the anterior sectors, from an aesthetic point of view we need space.

Framing a smile helps us clinicians avoid problems and allows the technician to work better. The questions to ask before we start are:

- Do I need to do ameloplasty on any tooth or can I proceed with additive-only techniques?
- Do I need to reposition the gingival parabolas?
- Do I have room for a proper midline?

Everything we plan carefully will lead us to simplify procedures and optimize the results with greater satisfaction for us and our patients.

SUGGESTED READINGS

- Coachman C, De Arbeola L, Mahn E. An Improved direct injection technique with flowable composites. A digital workflow case report. *Oper Dent.* 2020;45(3):235-242.
- Devoto W, Saracinelli M, Manauta J. Composite in everyday practice: how to choose the right material and simplify application techniques in the anterior teeth. *Eur J Esthet Dent.* 2010;5:102-124.
- Dietschi D. Optimizing smile composition and esthetics with resin composites and other conservative esthetic procedures. *Eur J Esthet Dent.* 2008;3(1):14-29.
- Hardan L, Bourgi R, Cuevas-Suárez CE et al. Novel Trends in Dental Color Match Using Different Shade Selection Methods: A Systematic Review and Meta-Analysis. *Materials.* 2022;15(2):468.
- Manauta J, Salat A. Layers. *An atlas of composite resin stratification.* Quintessence Publishing, 2012.
- Manauta J, Salat A, Devoto W, Putignano A. Layers 2. Direct Composites: *The styleitaliano clinical secrets.* Quintessence Publishing, 2022.
- Terry DA. *Restoring with flowables.* Quintessence Publishing, 2017.

MARCIN KRUPINSKI

Poland

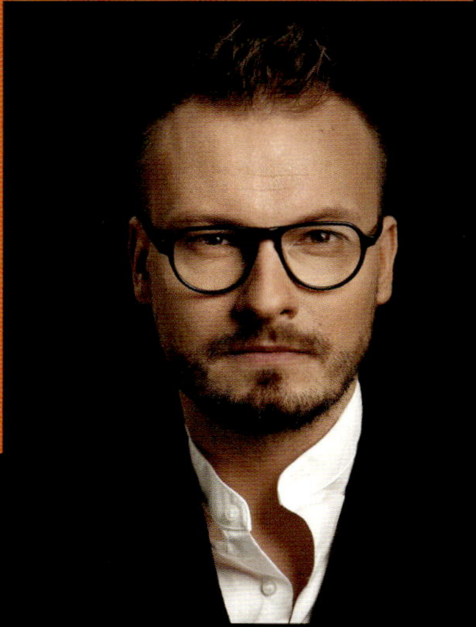

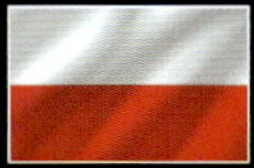

Marcin Krupinski graduated in Poland in 2010 from the Jagiellonian University Medical College in Krakow. From 2011-2014, he was an Assistant at the Department of Conservative Dentistry and Endodontics at the Jagiellonian University.
Winner of the Young Scientist Medal in 2011 for a clinical trial.
Key Opinion Leader for 3M/Solventum. Certified Trainer and Active Member of the StyleItaliano Group. He is the author of several publications and speaker in the field of restorative dentistry at numerous international conferences and workshops. Specialized in modern aesthetic dental treatment, he conducts his Private practice in Krakow, Poland.

BONDING WITH WAX-UP. HOW TO TRANSFER INFORMATION?

Aesthetics in the anterior region is no longer reserved only for composite masters. Thanks to new materials and simple step-by-step techniques, you can achieve a spectacular smile transformation in a single visit. Difficult cases are clinical situations where there is significant asymmetry, or the bite requires correction as well. In such situations, it is worth using the wax-up technique.

DISCUSSION AND CLINICAL CASE

A 24-year-old patient presented complaining about the aesthetics and asymmetry of her smile (📷 1). The patient was focused on achieving a brighter color but also symmetry was important. Due to her young age and generally healthy dentition, we decided on a non-invasive composite approach using bonding. Cases like this are difficult to achieve

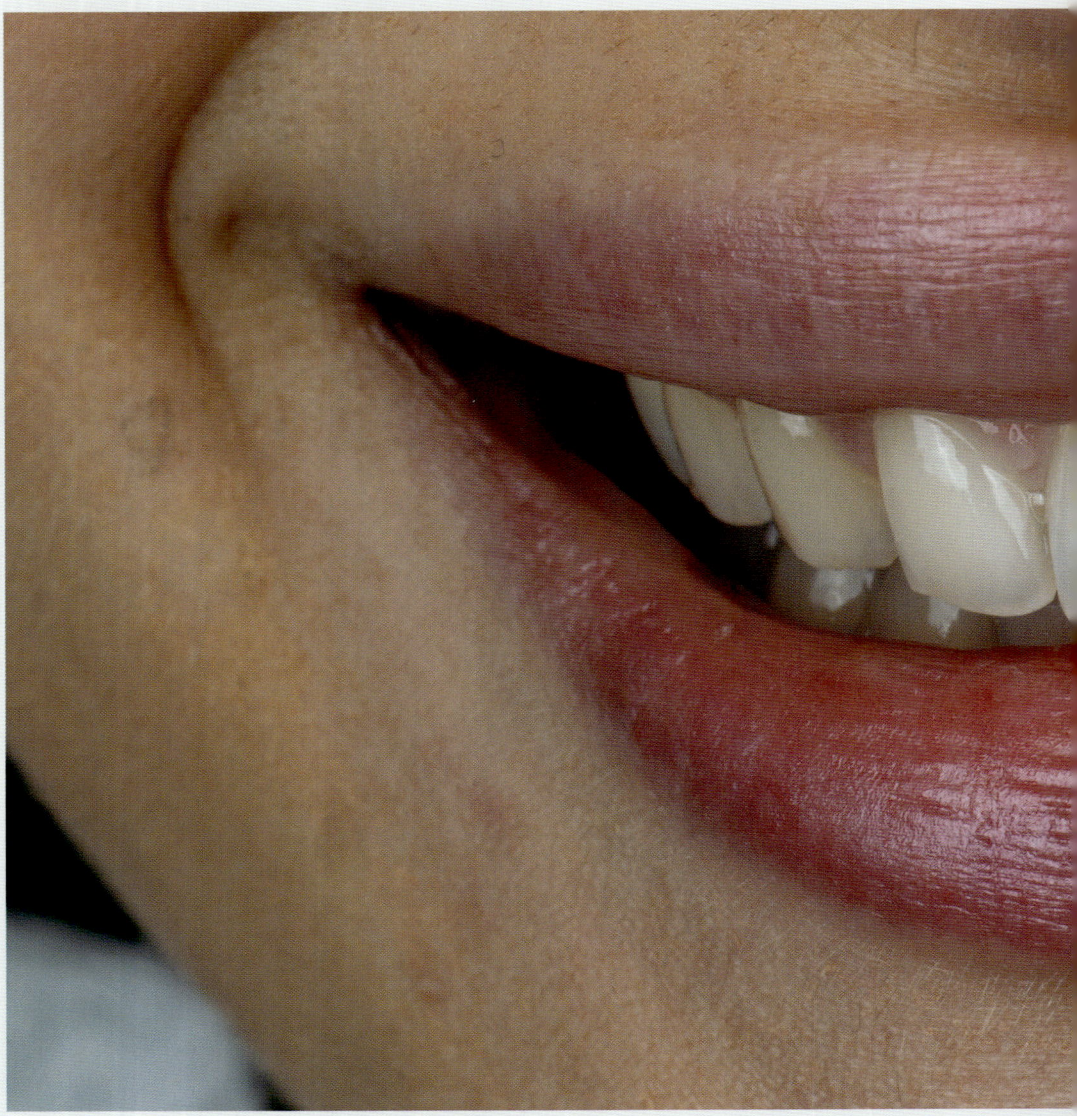

Figure 1 Initial situation of the patient. Visible asymmetry of teeth but rather healthy enamel.

with a direct approach. It is hard to achieve perfect symmetry and occlusal guidance with a free hand technique. That is why we always create a wax-up to test occlusion and outcome before procedure. There are several ways to copy wax-up information to the patient's mouth. This is one of the techniques for those clinical situations.

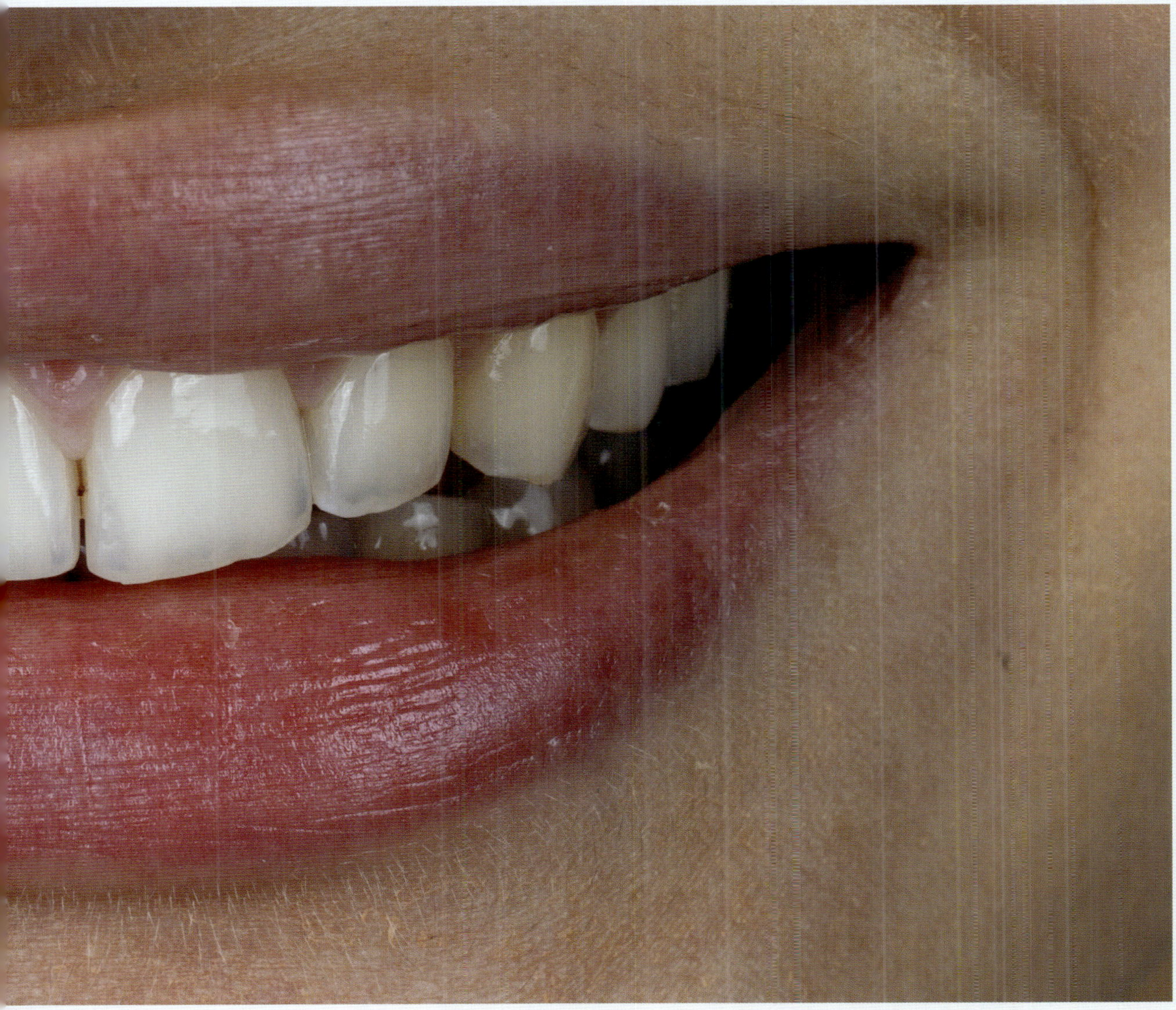

Preparation

For a "prepless" approach, we use the "split-dam" isolation, as with healthy periodontium and the technique presented, isolation is sufficient and non-damaging to the gums (📷 2). A transparent silicone mask based on the wax model was then 3D printed (📷 3); the vestibular portion was subsequently trimmed to avoid material ending up in the interproximal and cervical regions, where it is more difficult to remove and polish. These areas will be managed in a subsequent phase. Before bonding, the teeth were sand-blasted and etched, without enamel preparation. However, proper plaque and aprismatic enamel removal is crucial for the longevity of direct composite veneers. To facilitate the sandblasting phase and prevent bleeding, Lm Arte Gengiva can be used, which exposes the cervical area while simultaneously protecting the gums (📷 4).

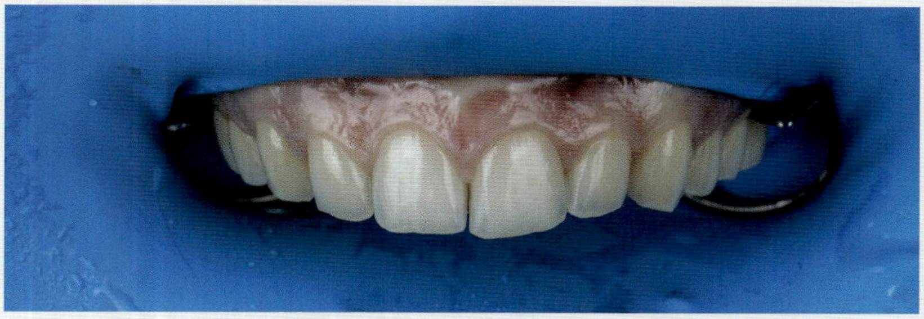

Figure 2 Isolation with split-dam technique. With proper periodontal health it is sufficient isolation for proposed technique and results in untouched gingiva at the end of procedure.

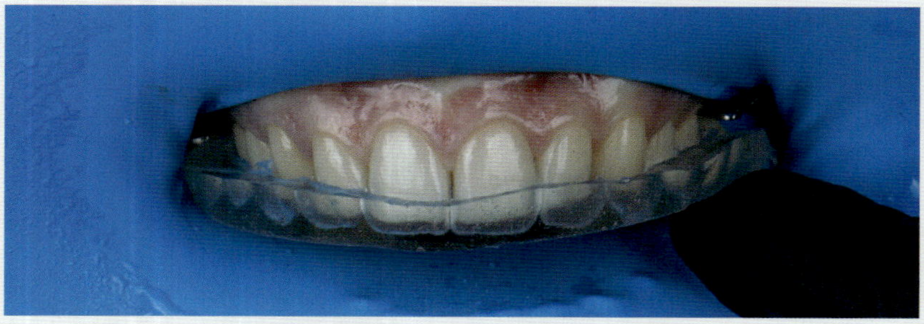

Figure 3 Transparent silicone index lets us copy wax-up for achieving symmetry and proper bite and guidance.

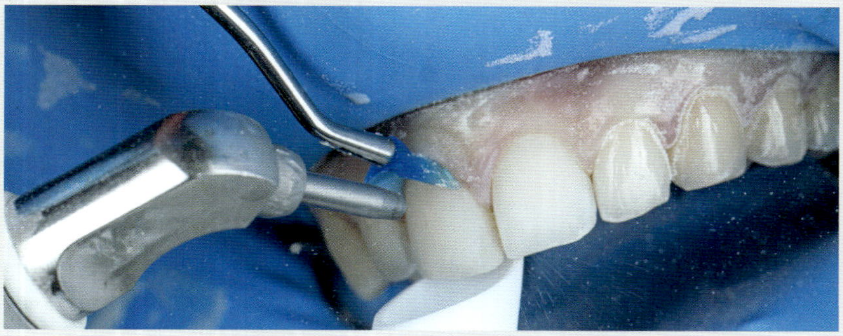

Figure 4 Sandblasting of enamel prior to adhesive steps helps remove biofilm and aprysmatic enamel, resulting in higher bond strengths. Lm Arte Gengiva helped to protect gingival margin.

Bonding

Following sandblasting and etching, we position the adhesive only on the incisal margins; this allows us to transfer information from the wax-up (5). When working with a monochromatic approach, we can obtain much more information from the wax-up than usual. Not only does it enable us to replicate the position and guidance of the incisal margins, but it also allows us to transfer information regarding the thickness of the direct veneers (6). At this point, we can trim the interproximal spaces since we currently do not need material there, which will be placed later (7). Therefore, thickness, symmetry, and positions of the incisal margins have been transferred. In the next phase, we can work with the Unica Anterior matrices (8). With these, we will achieve a smooth and compact composite in the interproximal and cervical areas, which are the most challenging for excess removal and polishing. With this approach, the vestibular surface is easy to fill, as if it were a large Class V restoration.

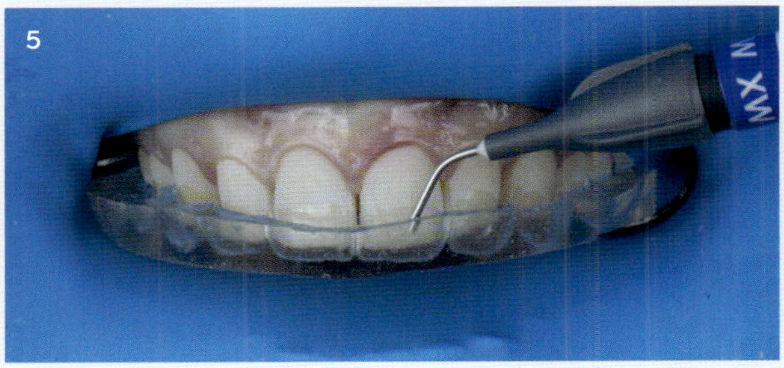

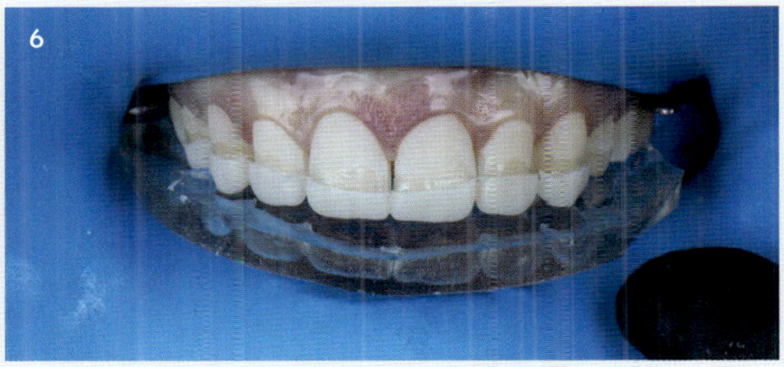

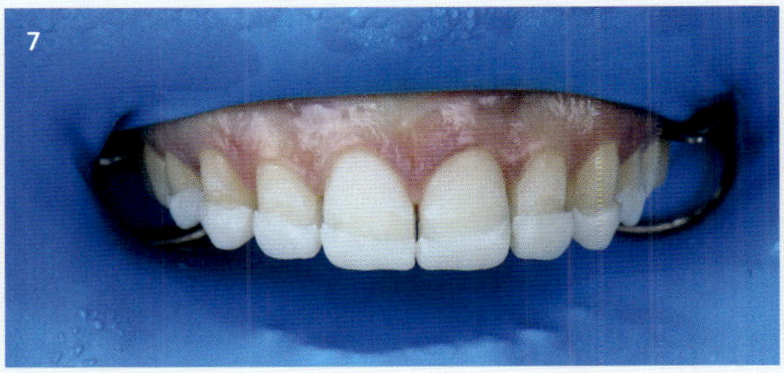

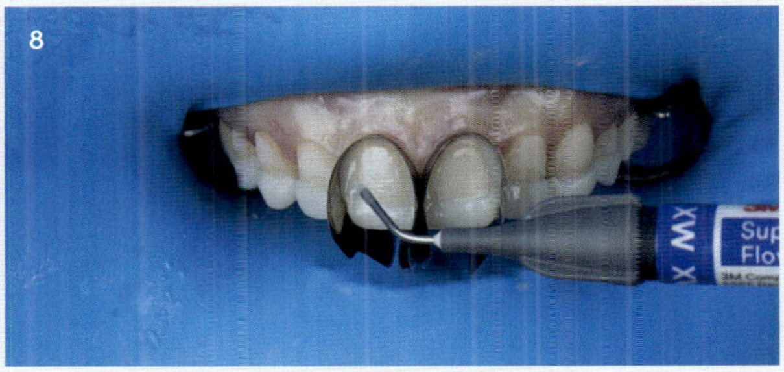

Figure 5 In the initial step only incisal margins are covered with adhesive and flowable composite is used in this case to copy edges and incisal guides from wax-up.

Figure 6 Usually, only the incisal margins are copied; however, in the proposed technique, since we are working with a single-mass composite, it is possible to replicate the vestibular portion as well.

Figure 7 The interproximals are cut for matrixes to be placed.

Figure 8 Then the Unica Anterior matrixes can be placed and labial surface can be filled with composite.

Shaping and finishing

After placing the composite using the Unica matrices, we move on to the modeling phase (📷 9). We use a SofLex coarse grit disc to remove excess material and provide a basic shape (📷 10). After shaping tooth by tooth, we follow the same steps for the rest of the smile (📷 11). Despite working with a single mass in this case, proper polishing and texturing will provide the patient with the desired natural smile (📷 12).

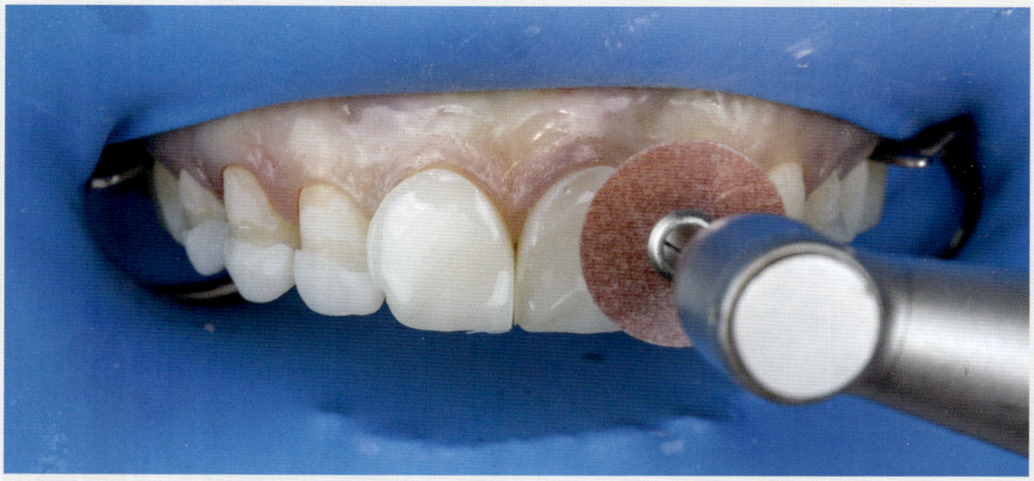

Figure 9 The composite was placed with excess. Now it is important to remove it and shape the future veneer.

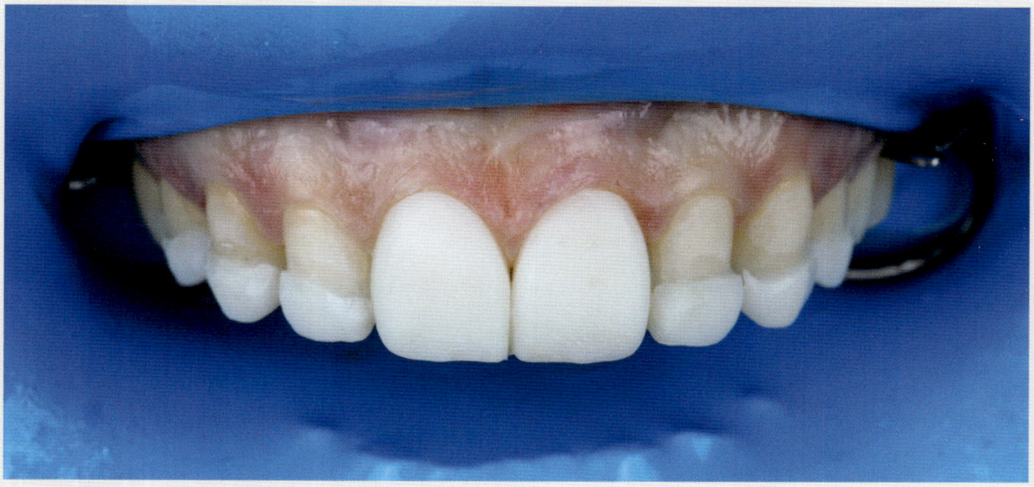

Figure 10 After achieving a basic shape we can check the symmetry of width and shape, and then proceed to the next tooth.

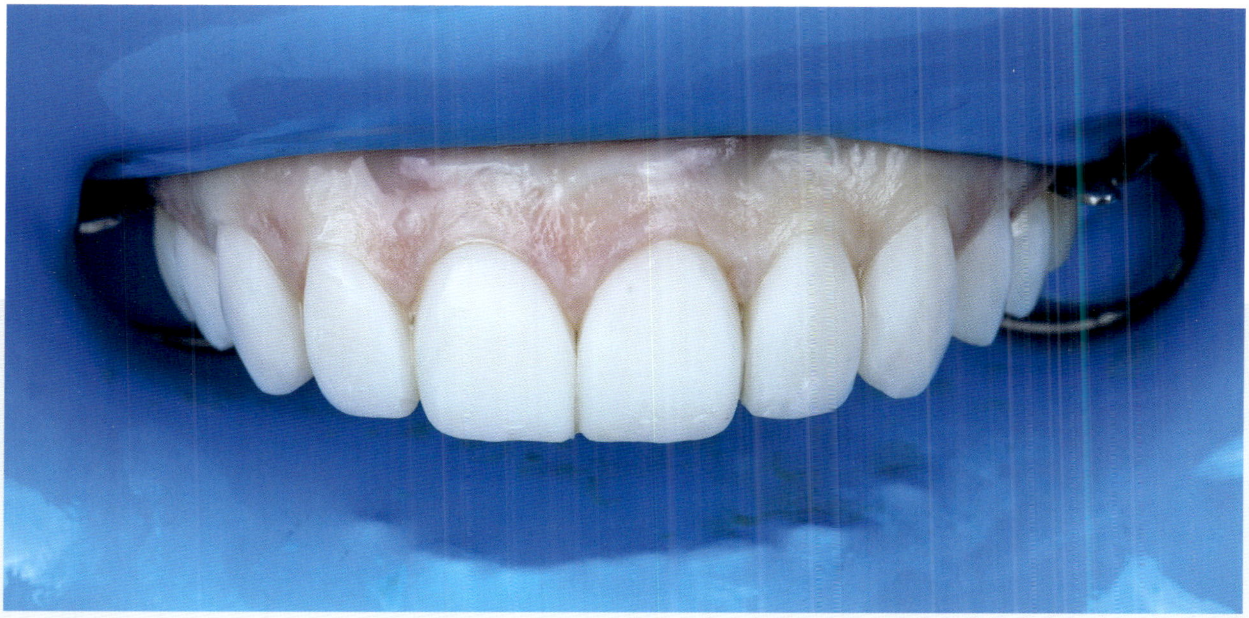

Figure 11 The same steps for rest of the teeth placing matrixes and composite with excess and shaping to the basic shape.

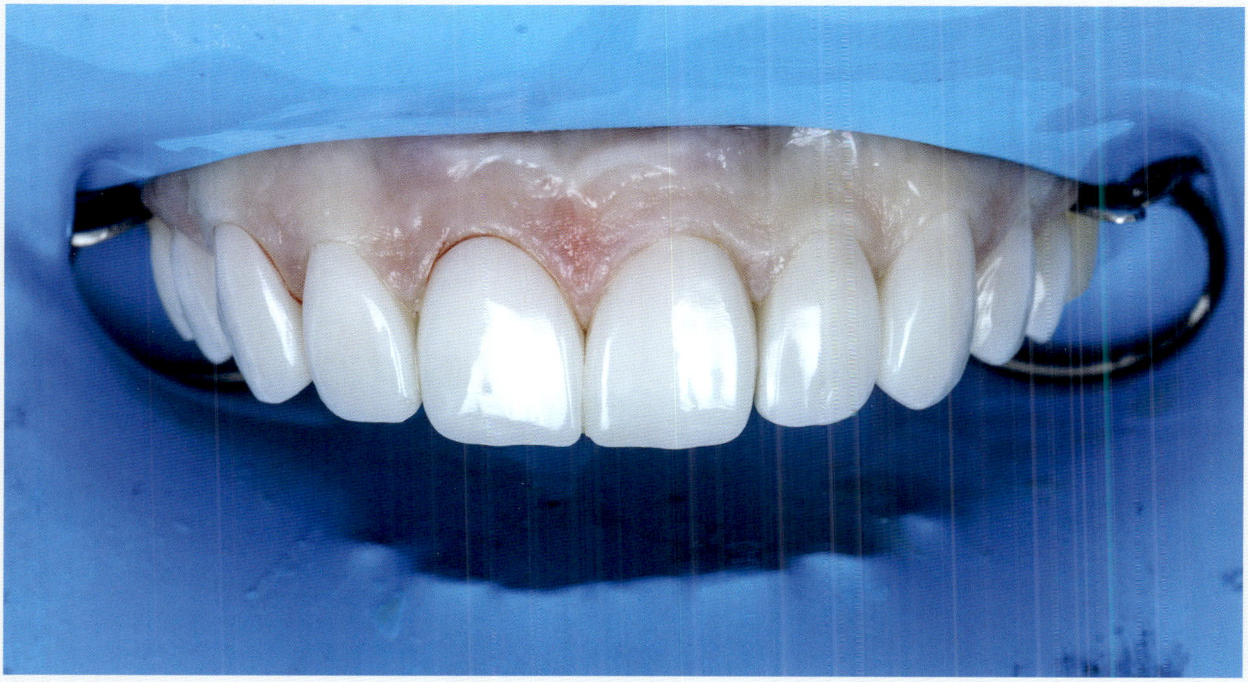

Figure 12 Even though it was done with a single shade, proper polish and texture provide a natural look.

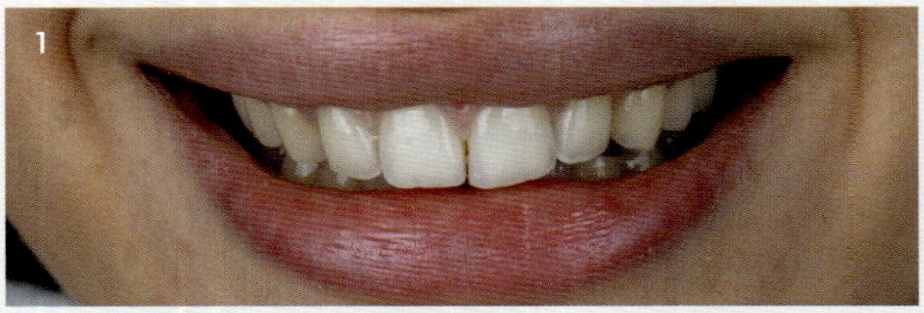

Figures 1, 13 Before and after. We see improvement of symmetry and shape of the teeth, with black spaces also being filled. The procedure was done completely without enamel preparation.

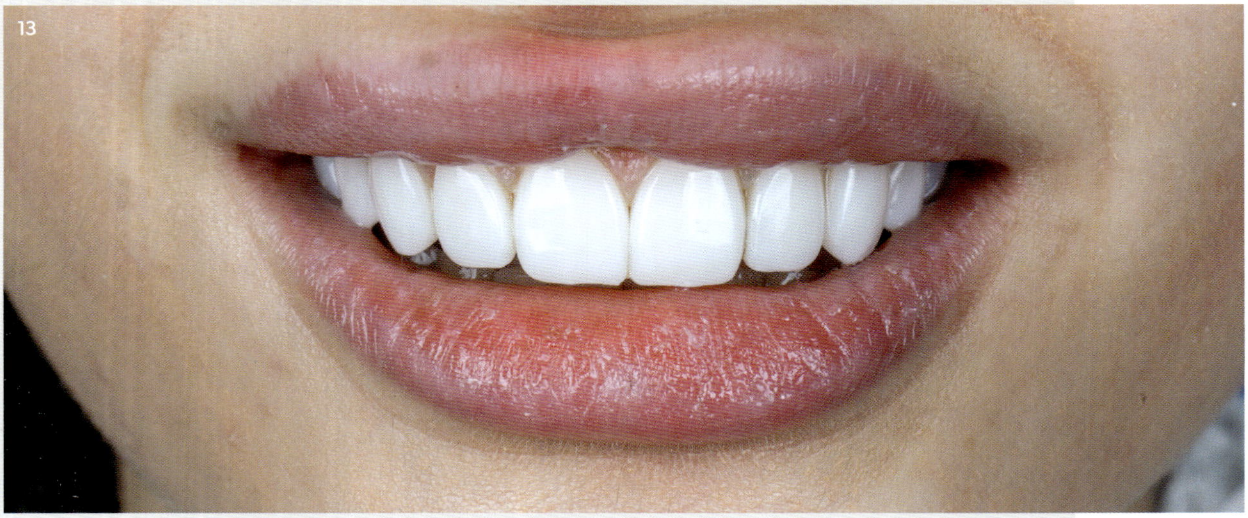

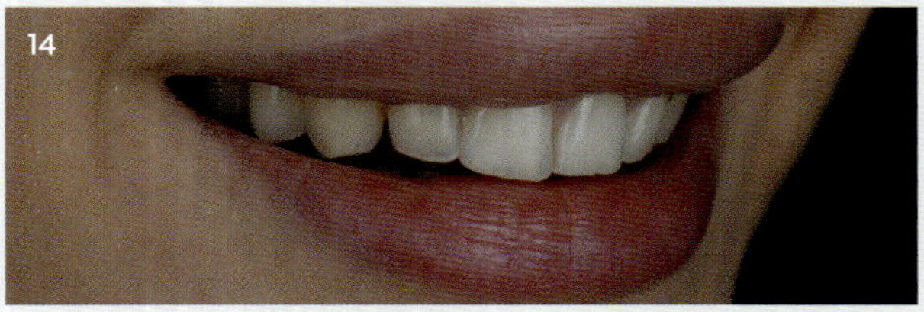

Figures 14, 15 Before and after. Despite working with a single shade when the shape and finish are appropriate, a natural look is achieved, giving great satisfaction to our patient.

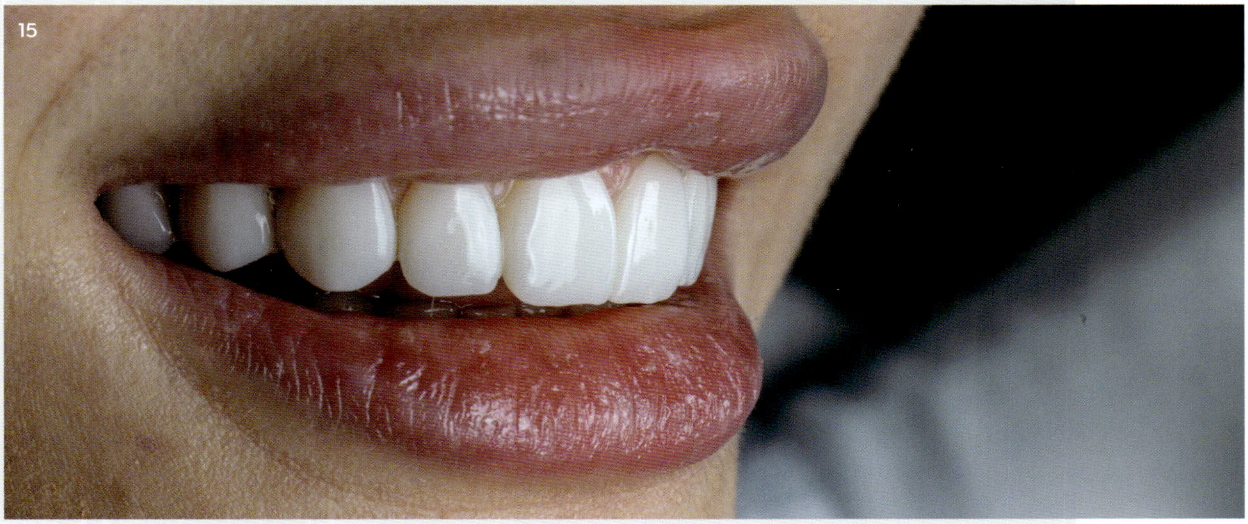

CONCLUSION

Transferring information from diagnostic wax-ups is crucial to achieving long-term results. In challenging cases like this, with asymmetries and occlusal problems, 1:1 transfer is crucial. When working with a single-mass composite, this step can be quick and lead to a satisfying outcome for our patient, while preserving functional appearance. The final smile can also be checked and adjusted to the patient's liking (📷 1, 13; 14, 15). Composite bonding can be a life-changing approach for both aesthetic and functional restorations, without requiring overly long and complicated procedures.

SUGGESTED READINGS

- Baldissera RA, Corrêa MB, Schuch HS et al. Are there universal restorative composites for anterior and posterior teeth? *J Dent.* 2013;41(11):1027-35.
- de Abreu JLB, Sampaio CS, Benalcázar Jalkh EB, Hirata R. Analysis of the color matching of universal resin composites in anterior restorations. *J Esthet Restor Dent.* 2021;33(2):269-276.
- Ghazal M, Albashaireh ZS, Kern M. Wear resistance of nanofilled composite resin and feldspathic ceramic artificial teeth. *J Prosthet Dent.* 2008;100(6):441-8.
- Goldstein RE. Universal composite resins: the "do-all" workhorses of dentistry... a system survey. *Dent Today.* 2005;24(2):150, 162, 164 passim.
- Manauta J, Salat A. Layers. *An atlas of composite resin stratification.* Quintessence Publishing, 2012.
- Monteiro P. Essential Shape. The key to a tooth-like restoration. *Styleitaliano.org*, 2020;7.
- Okeson JP. *Tooth Wear Management of Temporomandibular Disorders and Occlusion.* 6th ed. Mosby 2008;245-247.
- Vanini L, D'Arcangelo C. EFP. *Esthetics, function, posture.* Edra Publishing, 2024.

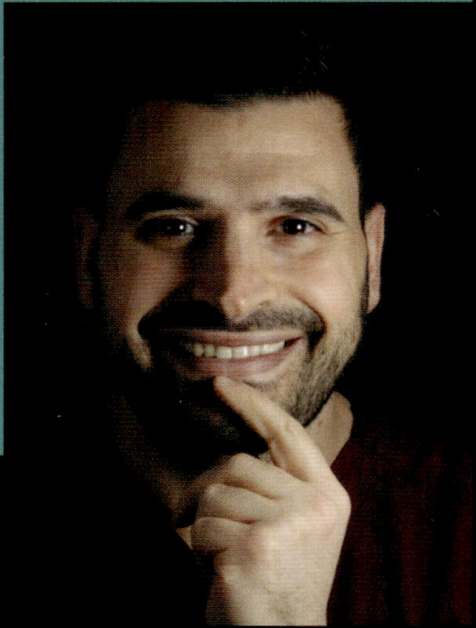

AHMED SAMER TADFI

United Kingdom

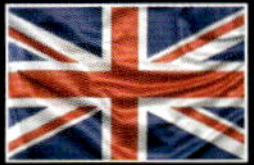

Having graduated from the University of Birmingham in 2014, Dr. Tadfi successfully completed his training program and now works at a private dental practice in London. At an early stage in his career, he lectured nationally and internationally.
He is a key opinion leader for several dental companies.
In 2018, he received numerous awards, including Best Young Dentist in the UK and, internationally, second prize in the StyleItaliano bulk contest.
He was also a finalist for the Private Dentistry Awards for Best Young Dentist in 2018.
Since 2019, he has been an active member of StyleItaliano.

PASTE-FLASK: A NEW CHAIRSIDE FRONTIER IN MODERN DENTISTRY

Restoring anterior teeth in a single session using high-quality modern composite is the desire of every dentist.
Achieving the "wow" effect on the patient, this provides a quick and cost-effective solution without requiring special artistic skills, utilizing a forgiving material that mimics the appearance of a ceramic restoration.
Now, achieving this goal is possible through a few techniques for using the available composites, and the simplifications developed and presented by StyleItaliano. One dentin shade and one enamel are sufficient to achieve a natural effect to achieve the desired outcome.
This article introduces an innovative technique that exploits the designs achievable in the lab, along with a set of tools that can significantly streamline on-patient work for the clinician. It is a technique accessible to all, aiming to serve and impress our patients.

DISCUSSION AND CLINICAL CASE

A 38-year-old patient visited expressing dissatisfaction with the upper anterior teeth, citing concerns about their shapes, discoloration, and signs of wear. The patient desired a slight improvement in color, specifying "not too much", and sought to achieve symmetry (📷 1-3). We suggested taking a scan and thoroughly studying the case with the intention of crafting appropriately shaped additive restorations, aligning them as accurately as possible.

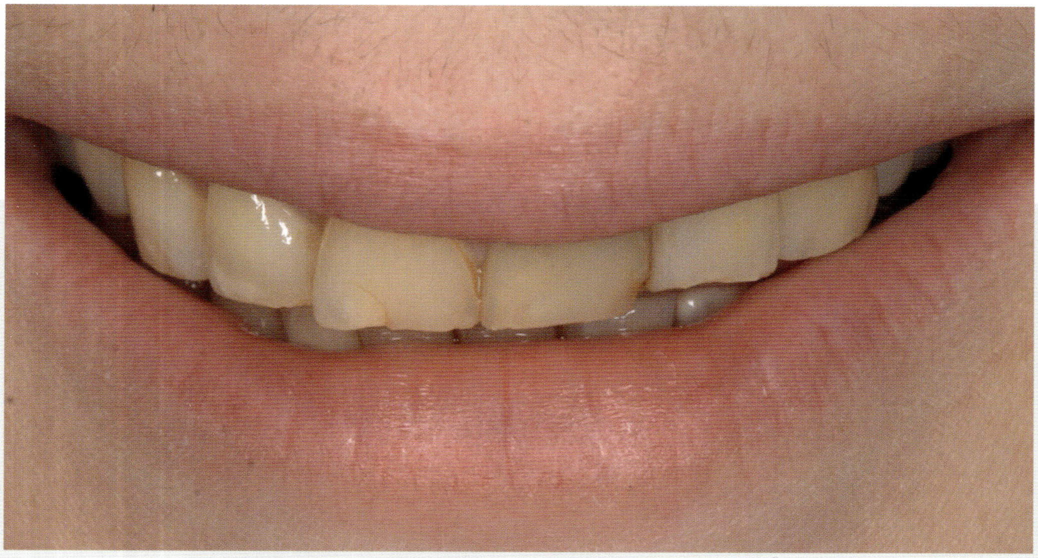

Figure 1 Initial patient smile.

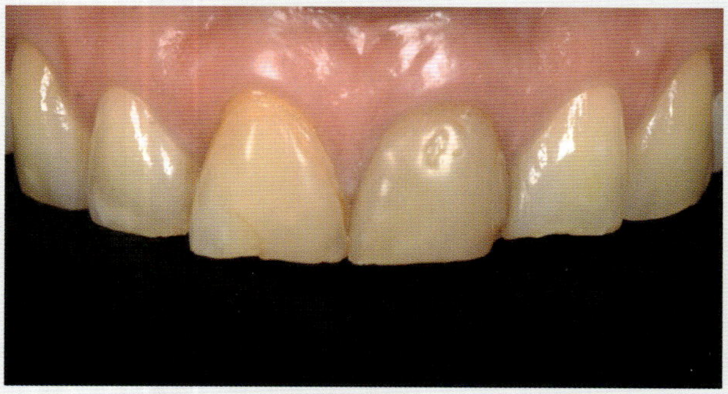

Figure 2 Initial situation. Note the asymmetrical appearance of the front 4 teeth and the altered gingival contours. In addition, we see some old composite material on the upper left central incisor.

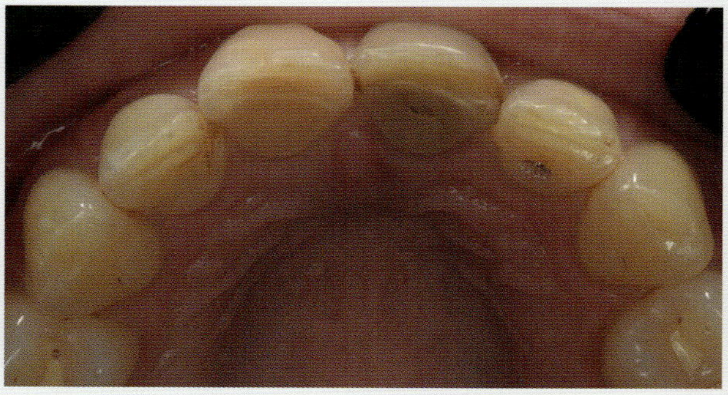

Figure 3 The occlusal view of the anterior group is the most important to set up an additive treatment plan usually following the profiles of the two canines.

In the laboratory, in collaboration with our dental technician, Mr. Daniele Rondoni, we were able to formulate a new design based on the scans **(📷 4-6)**.

In the subsequent session, the response to the mock-up left both us and the patient enthused **(📷 7)**. The aesthetics were excellent, entirely additive, and showcased a beautiful outcome, an achievement that is not straightforward, even with advanced direct techniques. Additionally, the gingival contours appeared optimal, allowing for a natural appearance of the entire smile.

Considering these positive outcomes, we suggested indirect composite restorations (veneers) to the patient, relying on our extensive experience with the quality and durability of such restorations. However, due to limited financial resources, the patient couldn't accept this proposal, leading us to explore an alternative solution. Since we already had the new smile designed and the silicone **(📷 8)** from the mock-up, the idea arose to directly apply composite onto the healthy teeth.

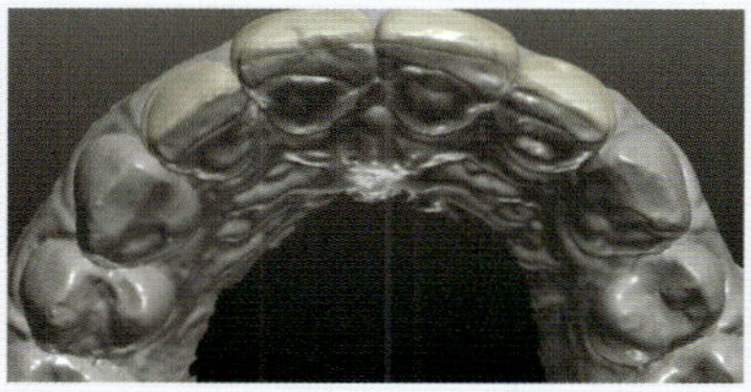

Figure 4 We proposed to take a scan and to study the case. Here we can see the proposed "addition" of restorative material.

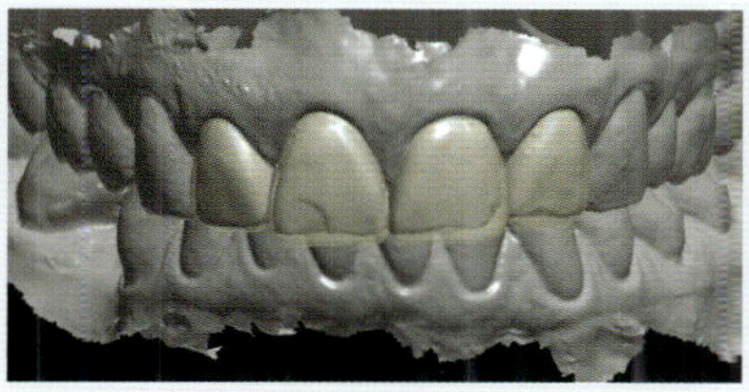

Figure 5 Again, from an anterior perspective the proposed addition of composite material.

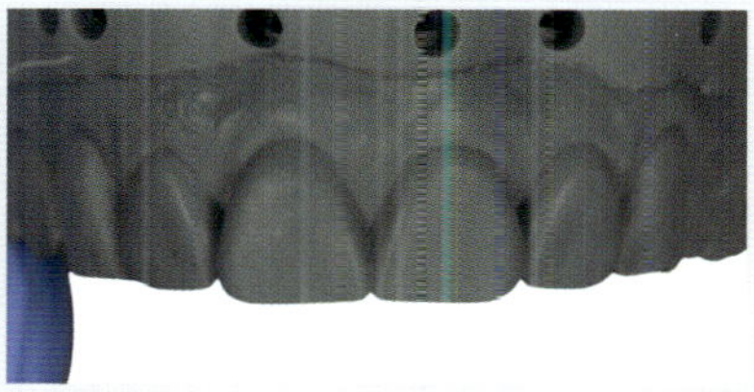

Figure 6 The 3D printed model to "preview" with the patient chairside. The technician can create a silicone putty for the dentist, or the dentist can choose to make one chairside also using this model.

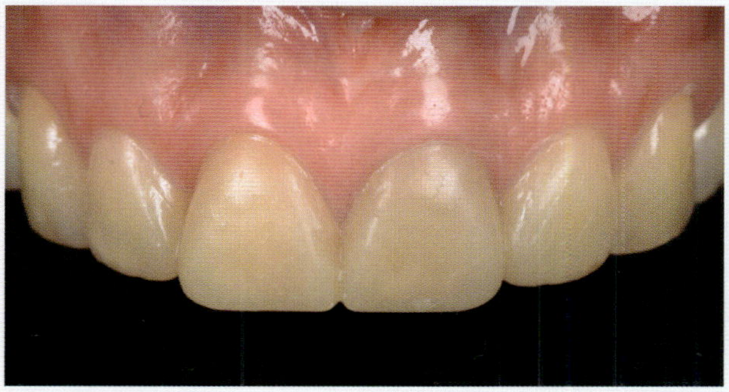

Figure 7 The mock-up directly transferred on to the patient using DMG Luxatemp material which helped the patient visualize the potential final outcome. The patient was very pleased to go ahead with this proposal.

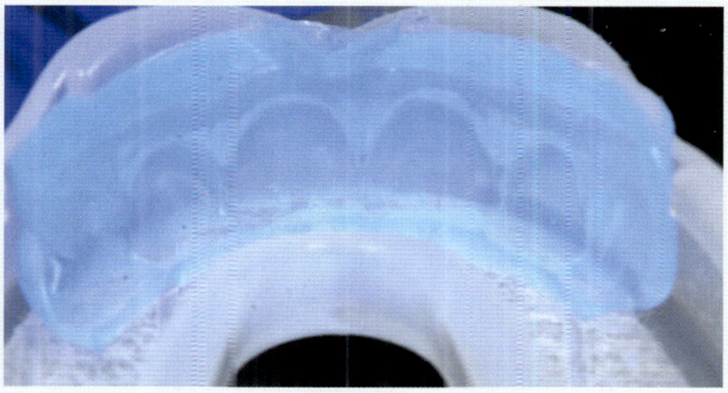

Figure 8 A transparent silicone index was taken from the 3D model in order to make the "semi-direct" composite restorations.

During the subsequent session, which lasted about 2 hours, we proceeded tooth by tooth as follows. The old composite on the upper left central incisor was removed and the any rough or sharp edges were polished off using the 3M Soflex disc **(📷 9)**. The teeth are then covered with a strip of Teflon tape **(📷 10)**. Universal shade composite was carefully placed into the silicone key using a suitable instrument (Modella, LM Arte by StyleItaliano), directed towards the incisal part **(📷 11)**. Subsequently, the silicone key was positioned on the selected tooth **(📷 12)**, applying slight pressure. Once the position was set, the composite was light-cured through the silicone key using a Curing Pen (Eighteeth) **(📷 13)**.

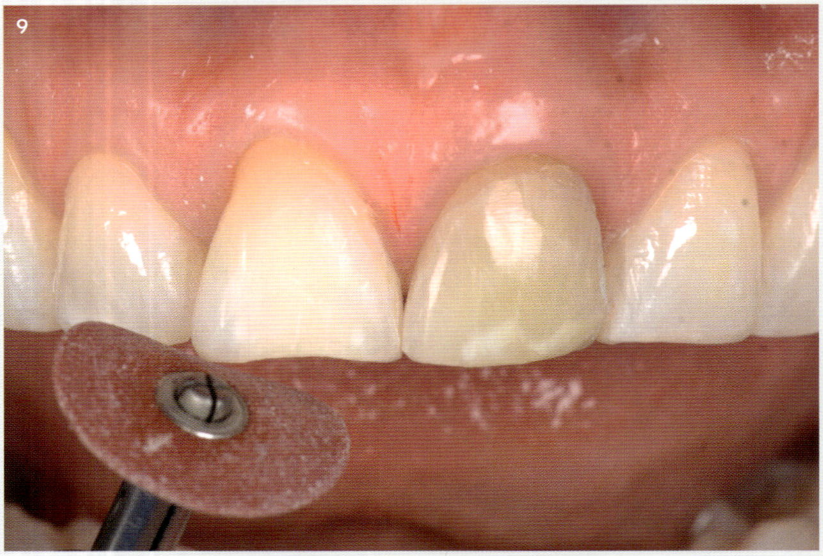

Figure 9 The teeth were cleaned, and the rough surfaces polished with a Soflex disc. The old layer of composite on the upper left 1 was also removed.

Figure 10 A strip of Teflon tape is applied to the teeth.

Figure 11 The composite used here was a universal shade and thus could be applied in one single mass. This limits the risks of introducing voids such as drags or air bubbles into the composite. It is worth noting that we can place the composite one tooth at a time or alternate teeth, i.e., UL1, UR2 and/or UR1 and UL2. This will help with efficiency and reduces time needed to make the composite veneers.

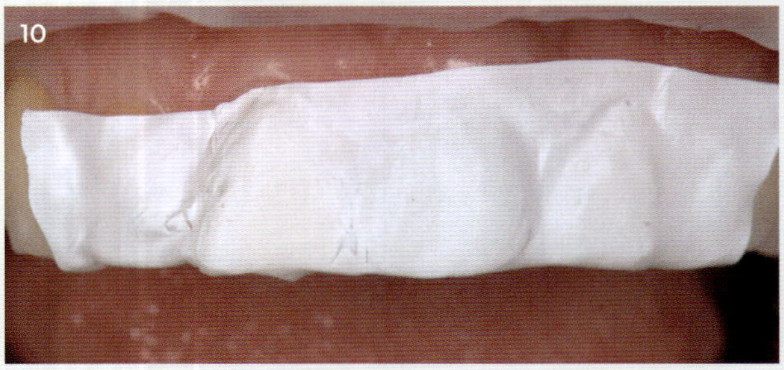

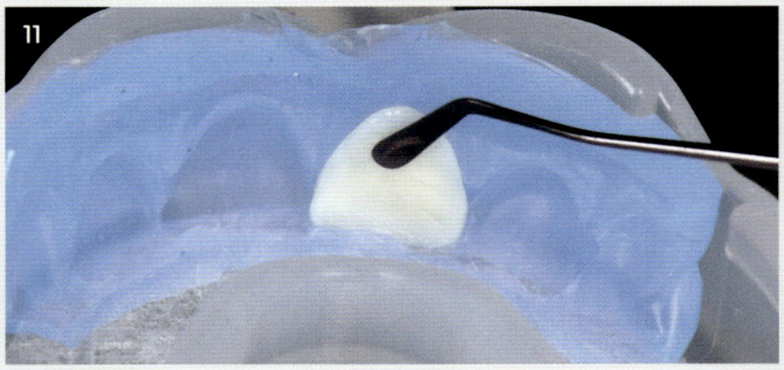

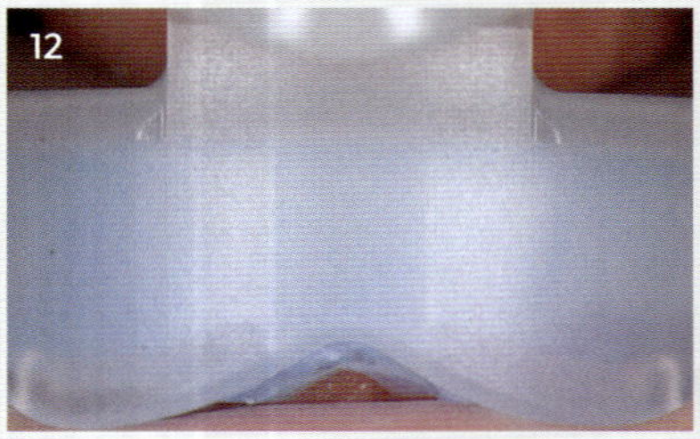

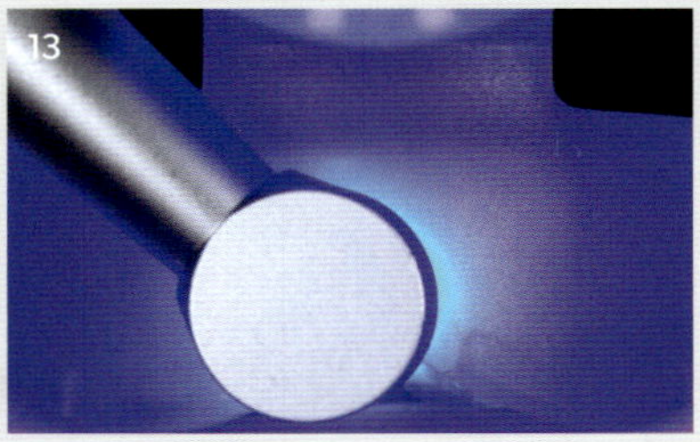

Figure 12 The silicone index is transferred onto the patient teeth and pressed well against the teeth ensure a constant pressure is applied for at least 10 seconds.

Figure 13 Whilst maintaining pressure the assistant then cures through the tray and silicone for 60 seconds.

After removing the key, the veneer seemingly appeared placed over the Teflon covered tooth (📷 14). Using an appropriate instrument (Arte Kit StyleItaliano, Fissura LM Co.), the veneer was gently taken off and refined outside the mouth (📷 15) (Kit Frese Finale StyleItaliano, Intensiv Co.). The outcome was thrilling. By repeating the same procedure for each tooth, it becomes feasible to individually isolate each tooth with the rubber dam and subsequently cement the veneers (📷 16).

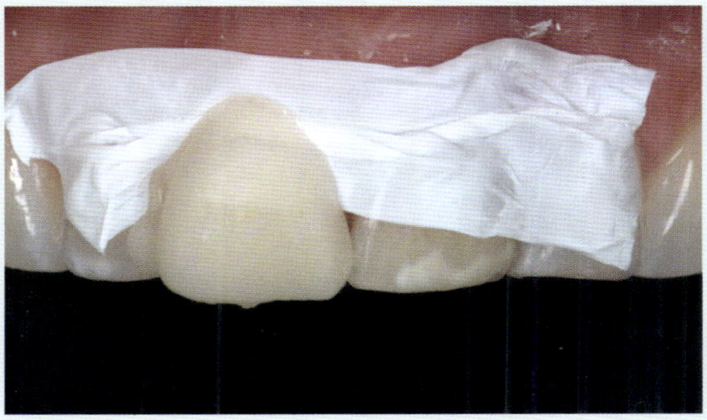

Figure 14 Remove the silicone index and cure once again for 30 seconds. Repeat this process until you have all the teeth you wish to restore.

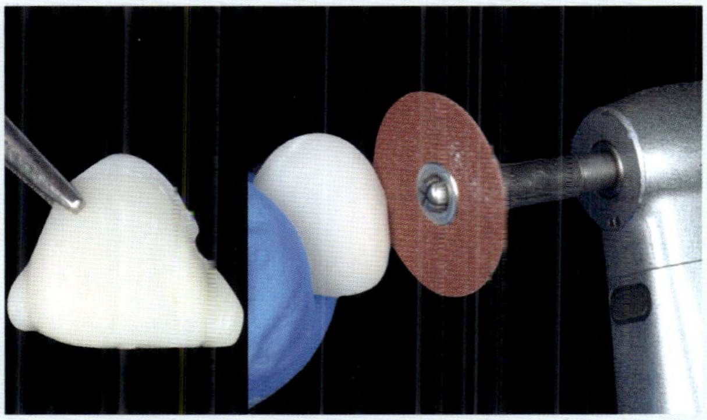

Figure 15 Now a Soflex disc or Optidisc can be used to trim back any excess composite material and refine the shape of the composite restoration if need be.

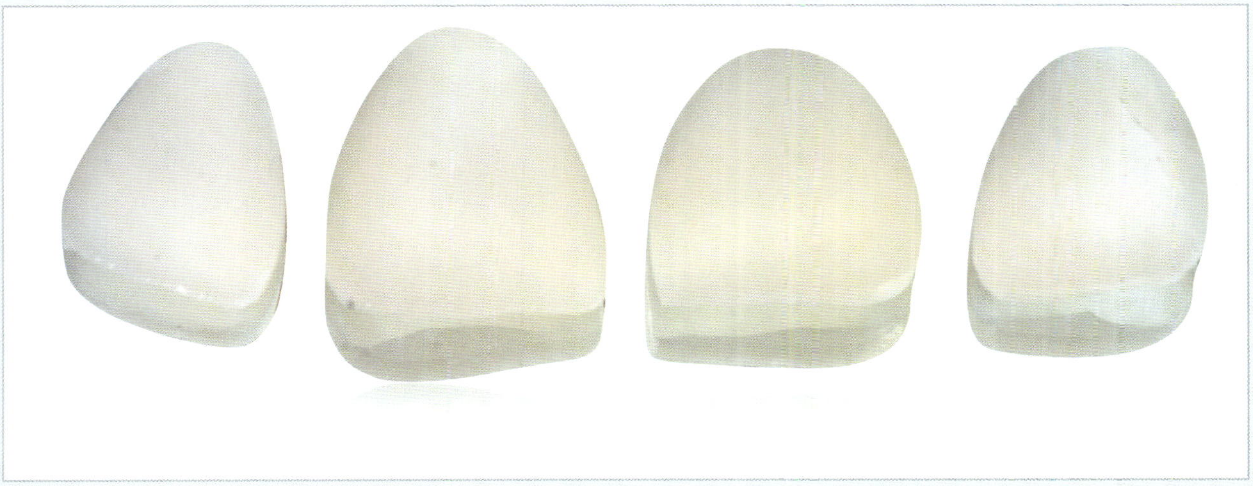

Figure 16 We now have the four "semi-direct" composite veneers ready for bonding.

This involves well-known steps: sandblasting (Air Flow Aquacare), phosphoric acid etching, adhesive application, veneer fitting, and cementation (17-20).

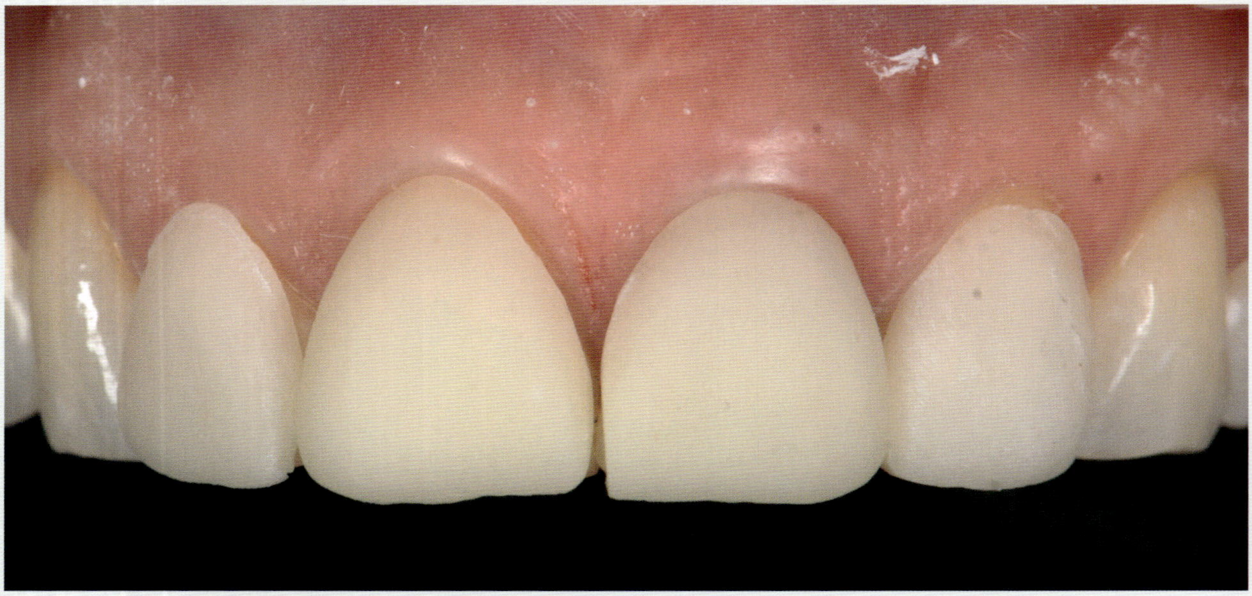

Figure 17 We should try the veneers on before starting the bonding process and before placing rubber dam. As we can see there are some small voids but overall the veneers fit well. The voids can be corrected during the cementation phase.

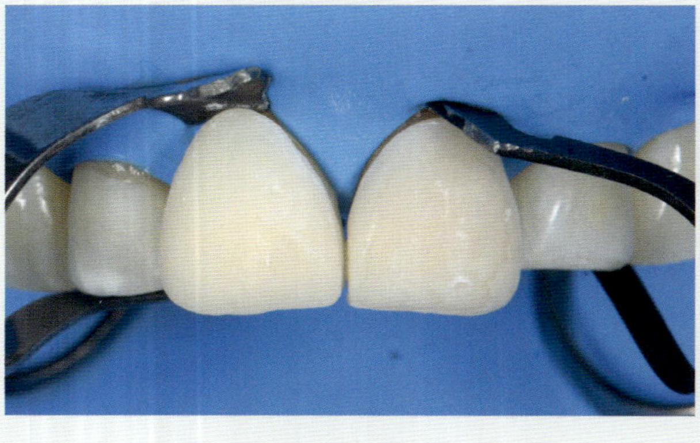

Figure 18 The rubber dam is placed and again the veneers are tried in for fit.

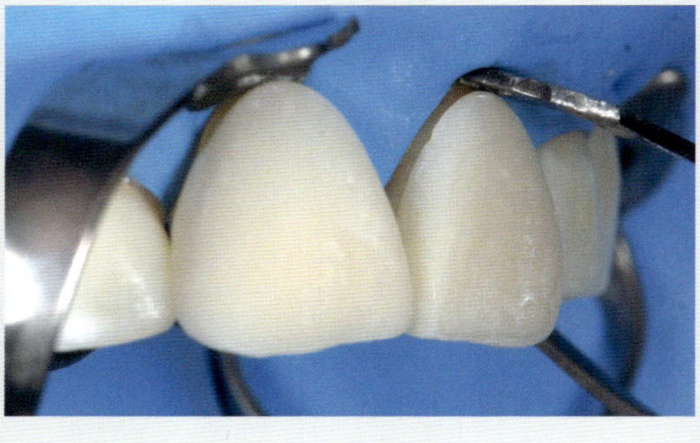

Figure 19 The fit of the composite veneers is good. Now the teeth are air abraded, etched using phosphoric acid, rinsed thoroughly, bonded and the veneers are cemented using wither a flowable composite or heated paste composite.

Following the adhesive procedures, the finishing touches on the veneers can be accomplished using a dedicated paste (Lucida, StyleItaliano), adhering to the steps to maintain the ideal shape and texture (21).

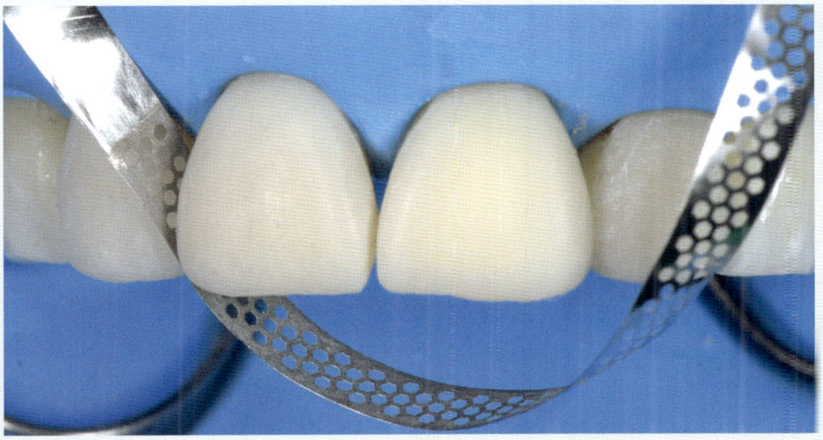

Figure 20 Once the veneers are cemented finishing and polishing strips may be used to remove any excess composite tags, bond, and flash.

Figure 21 A further enhanced polish using ASAP disc 2.

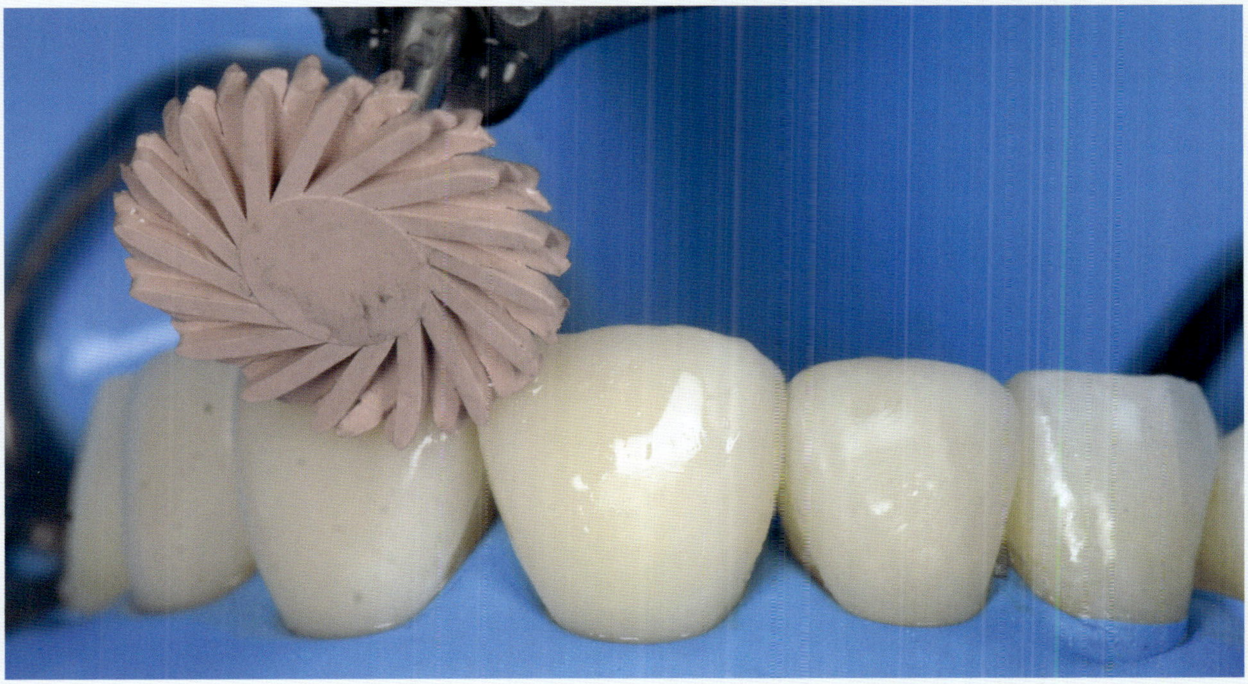

The ultimate outcome is highly satisfactory, given the simplicity of the suggested solution. Shape and color seamlessly blend within a brief chair time, without compromising the integrity of the sound dental structure. Moreover, the procedure allows for potential repairs and modifications at any time, all while maintaining a cost-effective approach for both the dentist and the patient (22, 23).

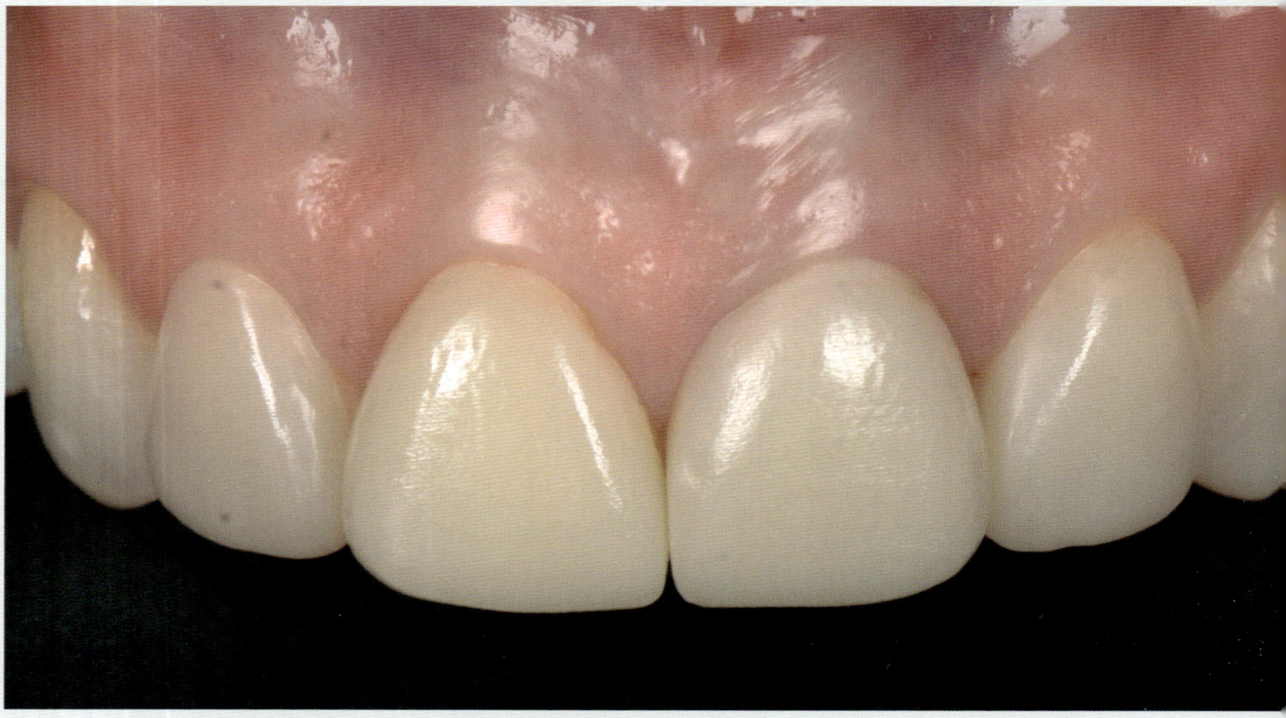

Figure 22 The patient returned one month later requesting some edge bonding on the canines to further enhance the smile and proportions, but we can see that the semi-direct veneers using the copy-flask technique have produced incredible results for the patient.

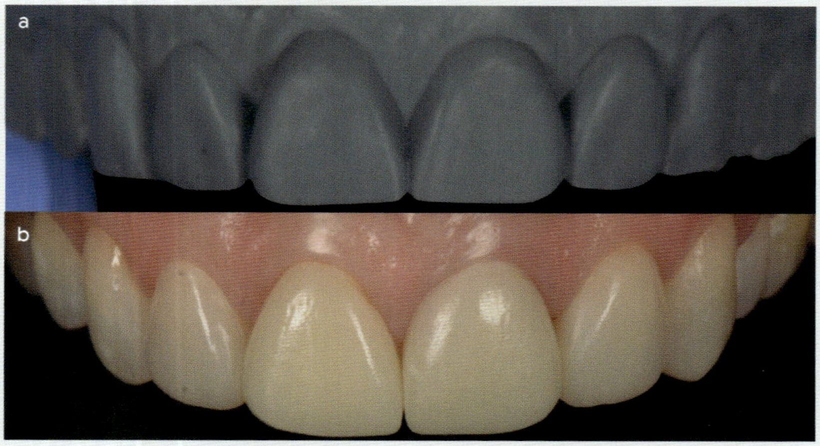

Figure 23 We can see how similar both the 3D printed model and outcome are when placed side by side for comparison.

CONCLUSION

Within the constraints of this approach, it presents a feasible solution for chairside restorations in situations where a prompt, aesthetically pleasing, adaptable, and repairable remedy is needed. It is particularly well-suited for both young and elderly patients facing financial constraints. Digital planning is easily accessible for modern dentists and proves highly beneficial in addressing restorative challenges in the anterior region, presenting the clinician and patient with an achievable outcome for aesthetic discussions. Composite is the preferred material for this technique due to its versatility, stability, and aesthetic qualities, even when using only two shades. In this scenario, the use of flowable materials, which tend to be fragile and exhibit diminishing aesthetics over time, is unnecessary. Similarly, there is no need to heat the paste composite, risking alteration of its intrinsic qualities.

In essence, this technique is user-friendly, accessible to dentists worldwide, and embodies the distinctive StyleItaliano approach.

SUGGESTED READINGS

- Devoto W. Direct and indirect composite restorations in the anterior area: a comparison between the procedures. *2QDT Yearbook*. 2003.
- Devoto W, Saracinelli M, Manauta J. Composite in everyday dentistry: How to choose the right material and simplify application techniques in the anterior teeth. *Eur J Esthet Dent*. 2010;5(1):102-124.
- Devoto W, Vanini L. Rifinitura e lucidatura dei restauri in composito. *Il Dentista Moderno*. 1999.
- Hardan L, Bourgi R, Cuevas-Suarez CE et al. Effect of different application modalities on the bonding performance of adhesive systems to dentin; a systematic review and meta-analysis. *Cells*. 2023;12(1):190.
- Magne P, Douglas WH. Additive contour of porcelain veneers: a key element in enamel preservation, adhesion, and esthetics for aging dentition. *J Adhes Dent*. 1999;1(1):81-92.
- Manauta J, Devoto W, Putignano A. I restauri del terzo cervicale: le problematiche dell'interfaccia digitale. *Dental Cadmos*. 2014;82(6):447-451.
- Manauta J, Paolone G, Devoto W. IN 'n' OUT – A New Concept in Composite Stratification. *Labline Magazine*. 2013;3(2):110-127.
- Manauta J, Salat A, Monterubbianesi R et al. Advances in diastema closure ans tooth shape change using direct restorations: the Front Wing Technique. *Int J Esthet Dent*. 2022;17(4):373-393.
- Paolone G, Orsini G, Manauta J. Composite shade guides and color matching. *Int J Esthet Dent*. 2014;9(2):164-182.

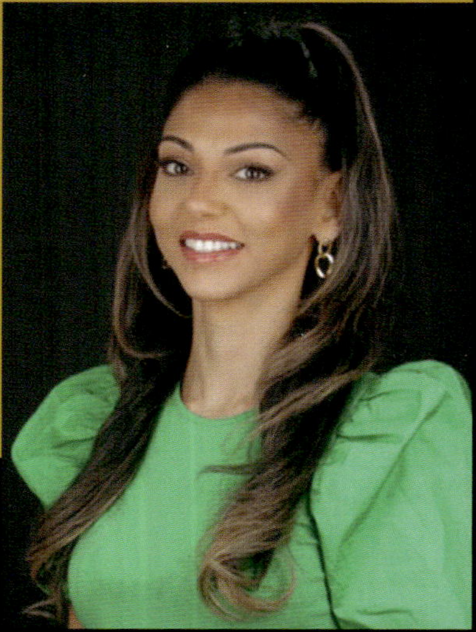

MEENAL PATEL

United Kingdom

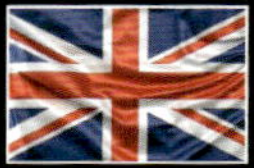

Meenal is a highly accomplished private general dentist specializing in smile makeovers and advanced restorative dentistry. Based in London and Surrey, she excels in handling complex restorative cases, transforming countless smiles.

With expertise in general and cosmetic dentistry, as well as facial aesthetics, Dr. Patel graduated with Honors from Bart's and The London School of Dentistry in 2012 and earned her BSc Honors in Pharmacology from King's College London in 2008.

Committed to continuous improvement, she has completed numerous international postgraduate training courses in Advanced Restorative and Cosmetic Dentistry. She stays at the forefront of her field through regular attendance at lectures and hands-on courses.

As a national lecturer in aesthetic dentistry, Dr. Patel conducts hands-on courses across the UK and showcases live case demonstrations in surgery. Recognized as a "Center of Excellence" for composite smile makeovers, she is among the top 20 centers

STYLOSO: GUIDANCE WITH LOVE

When direct composite may not be the most suitable treatment choice, and the patient cannot afford ceramics, it is important to consider and better understand the potential of indirect composite. The evolution of CAD-CAM digital technology has allowed the development of new techniques using innovative materials to plan and deliver smile makeovers using laboratory-milled composite veneers in a process known as Styloso.
Styloso is completed in a single-visit appointment saving significant chair-time, using 3D printed guides to facilitate only very minimal tooth reduction where necessary. Using a simple 2-plane reduction technique, we can deliver ceramic-like smile makeovers which are not only less destructive than a traditional veneer preparation, but less stressful and complicated for the dentist too.
The forgiving nature of composite allows us to quickly repair, refresh, adapt or modify it, at any time with limited expenditure for both the patient and dentist. The primary objective is to restore tooth structure while minimizing enamel loss during preparation. This is accomplished by providing reduction guides and precise veneers based on comprehensive digital planning, ensuring accuracy and efficiency in the process.

WHAT IS STYLOSO?

Styloso goes beyond being just a guided preparation technique focused on time efficiency. It represents a fundamental shift in our approach to minimally invasive preparation, striving for excellence in both aesthetics and long-term clinical outcomes.
Styloso represents an innovative approach to conservative tooth preparation, involving a 2-plane reduction process. The reduction takes place on the same day as bonding the veneers, with the assistance of 3D printed guides. By utilizing composite for both veneer and reline cement, a considerably stronger monolithic restoration is achieved, surpassing the outcomes of a direct technique. Indirect milled composite proves to be a superior and forgiving material, offering enhanced longevity, superior aesthetics, and the potential for future corrections.

The 2-plane reduction

The foundation lies in grasping the benefits of the 2-plane reduction, which not only preserves crucial tooth enamel but also lessens the stress and complications associated with veneer preparation. Reduced preparation using the 2-plane technique safeguards crucial cervical enamel. Unlike ceramic veneers that necessitate around 0.7 mm thickness for strength, often leading to preparation into the dentine at the cervical region, milled composite veneers present a distinct advantage with their unique properties requiring less preparation.
Following the curing process, composite veneers and the composite reline material seamlessly merge into a single strong monolithic restoration, ensuring robust margins despite the knife-edge finish. In contrast, ceramics demand a specific thickness at the margins to uphold structural integrity, hence requiring more extensive tooth preparation. By using a digital process, we can be less invasive and more predictable in our preparation planning.

DISCUSSION AND CLINICAL CASE

A 35-year-old female patient expressed concerns about the appearance of her teeth, specifically the irregular shapes, small size, and flat appearance **(1, 2)**. She hoped for a fuller smile to enhance her lip support and create a more youthful look, while expressing a desire to maintain the diastema, as it was a unique feature she wanted to preserve.

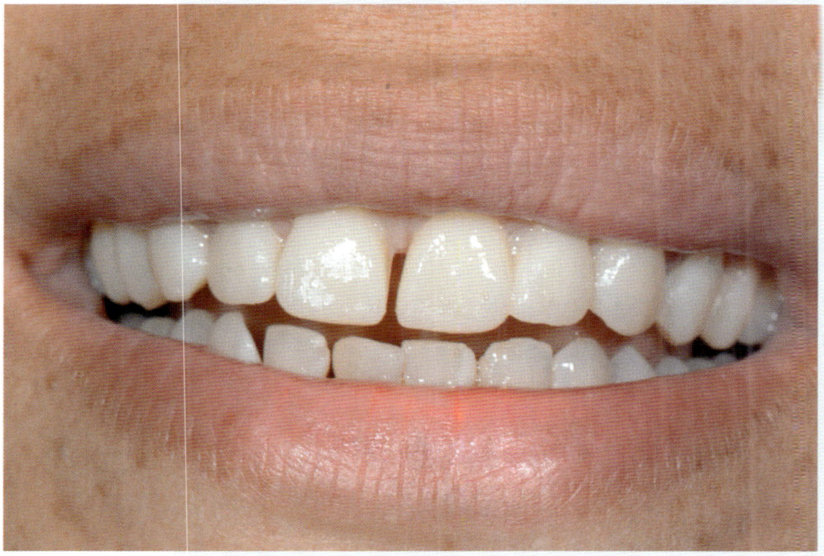

Figure 1 The initial smile with irregular incisal edges and shapes.

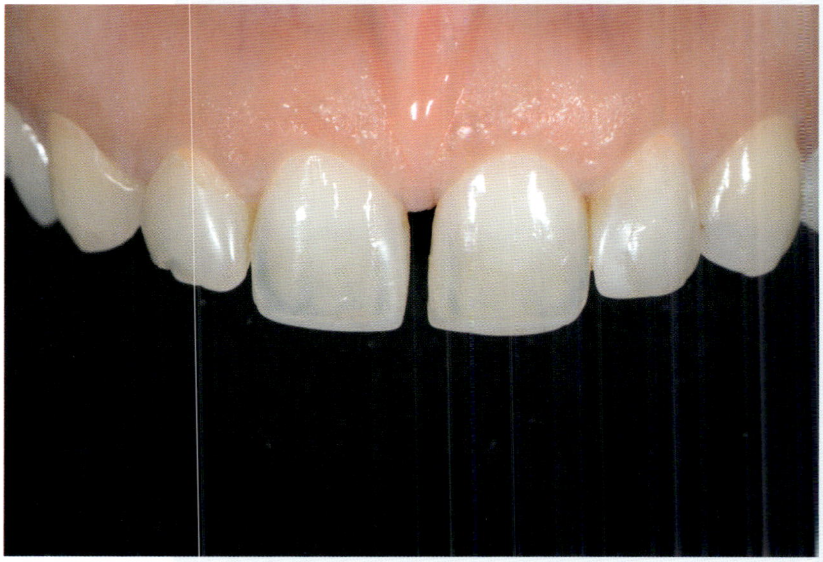

Figure 2 Retracted view of the initial situation. Note the flattened appearance of the central incisors due to tooth wear and irregular sizes of the lateral incisors.

A scan was taken and sent to the laboratory to create a digital wax-up for additive composite veneers (3-5). Through this digital process, the laboratory technician offers insights on the required incisal and vestibular preparation (6, 7).

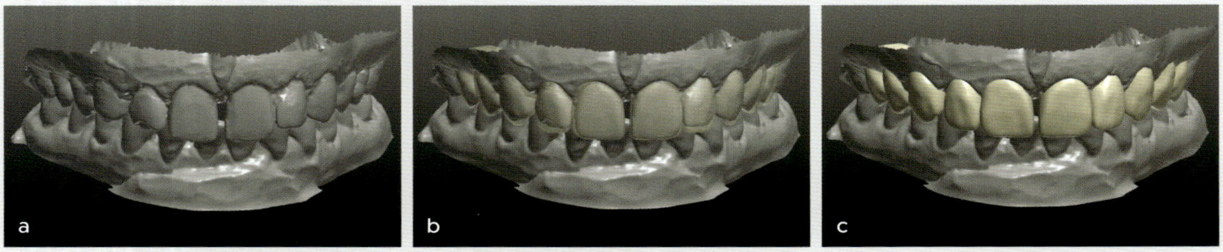

Figure 3 Previews of the digital smile design sent from the laboratory for 10 additive composite veneers. (a) The pre-operative scan. (b) The proposed design overlaying the original smile. (c) The final design.

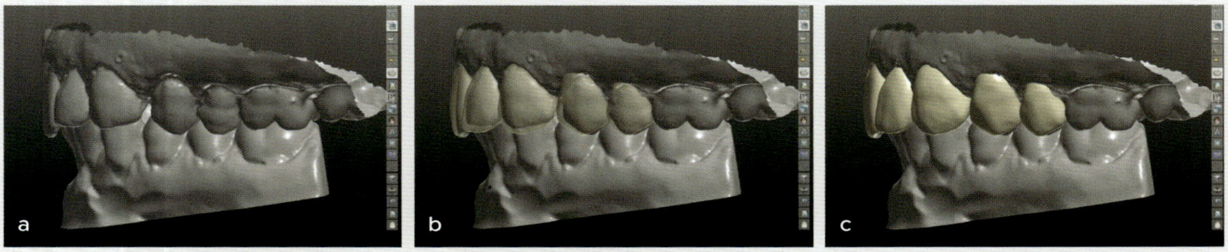

Figure 4 (a) Lateral view of the initial scan, (b) overlaid design and (c) final design.

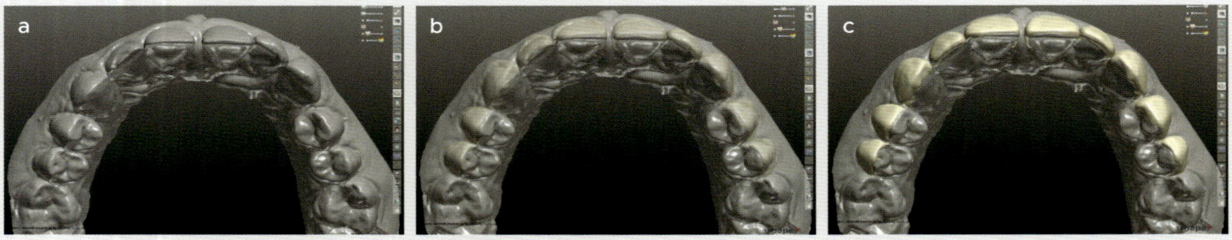

Figure 5 Occlusal view. (a) Initial situation. Note the thin volume of vestibular tooth tissue. (b) Proposed design overlaying the initial situation showing the increase in volume and additive approach. (c) The final design for additive composite veneers.

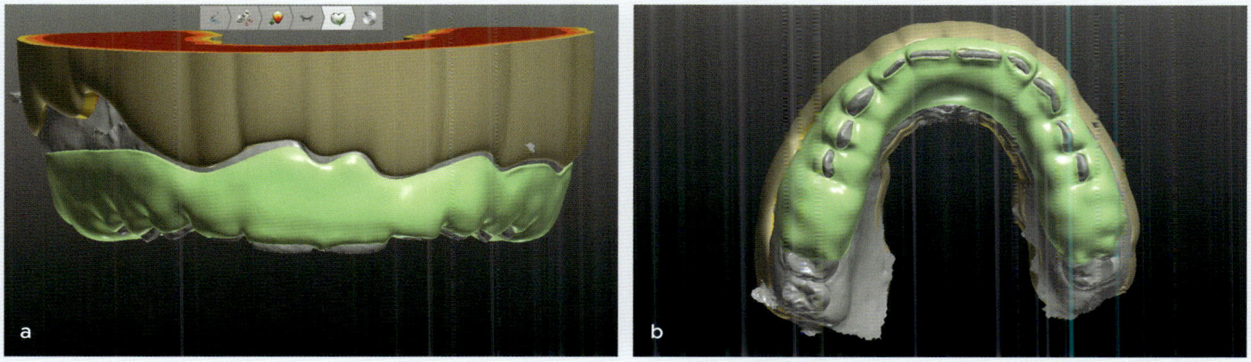

Figure 6 (a) A screenshot sent from the laboratory indicating the amount of incisal preparation and (b) a preview of the incisal preparation guide to be 3D printed.

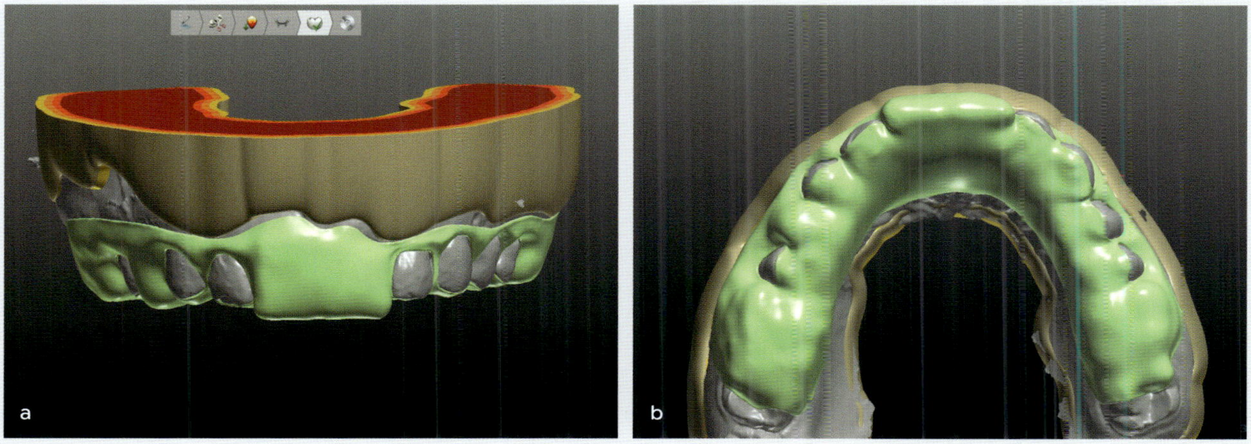

Figure 7 (a) The indication of the amount of vestibular preparation planned and (b) the preparation guide. Note there is no preparation of the central incisors or upper right premolar.

A 3D printed model and putty index of the smile design was created which allowed the patient to preview and trial their new smile in temporary acrylic material **(📷 8-10)**. Once we confirmed that the new design met the patient's esthetic goals, 3D printed reduction guides were created **(📷 11-15)** and the indirect composite veneers were milled in the laboratory **(📷 16)**.

The patient returned for their single-visit appointment in which the following steps were carried out.

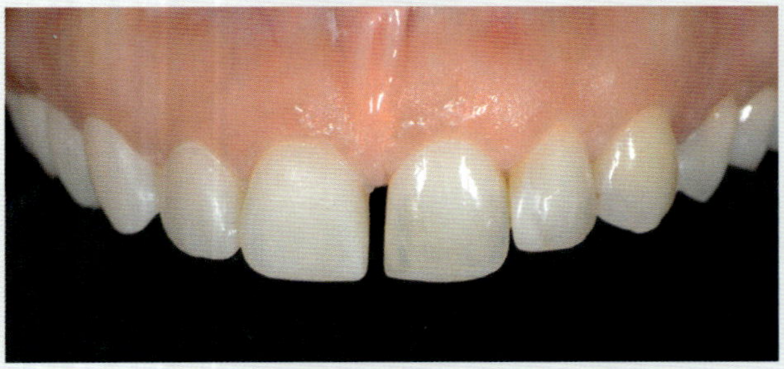

Figure 8 The trialed design is showcased on the left, while the initial situation is displayed on the right, enabling a comparison of the increase in volume and improvement in shapes.

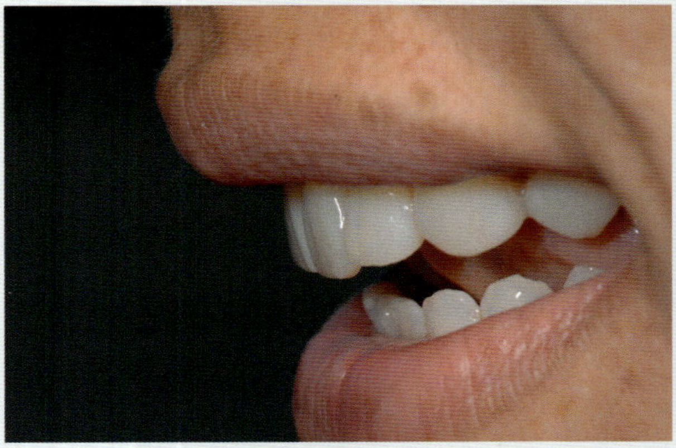

Figure 9 The side profile of the smile trial showing an increase in volume and improved lip support.

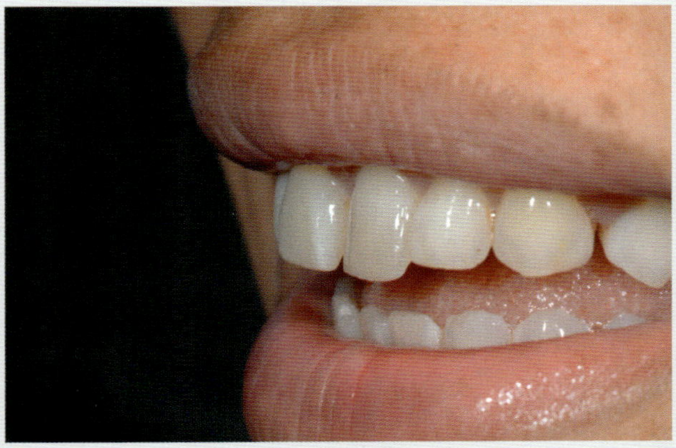

Figure 10 The side profile with the trial on the patient's right demonstrates that the proposal is primarily additive.

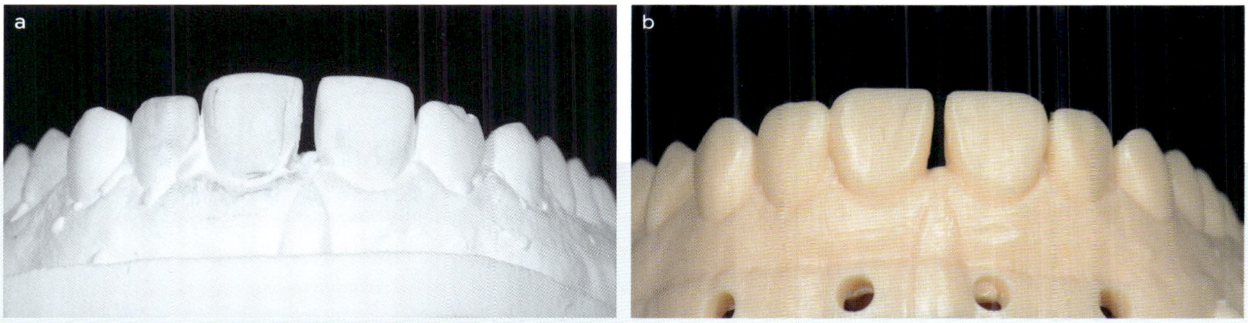

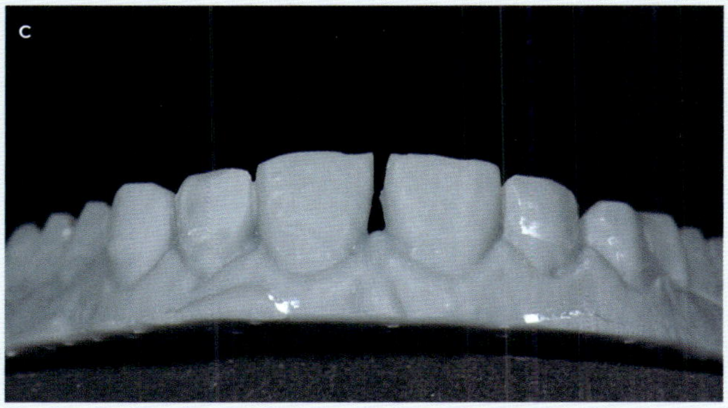

Figure 11 The models of (a) the original situation (b) digital wax-up design and (c) the prepared model.

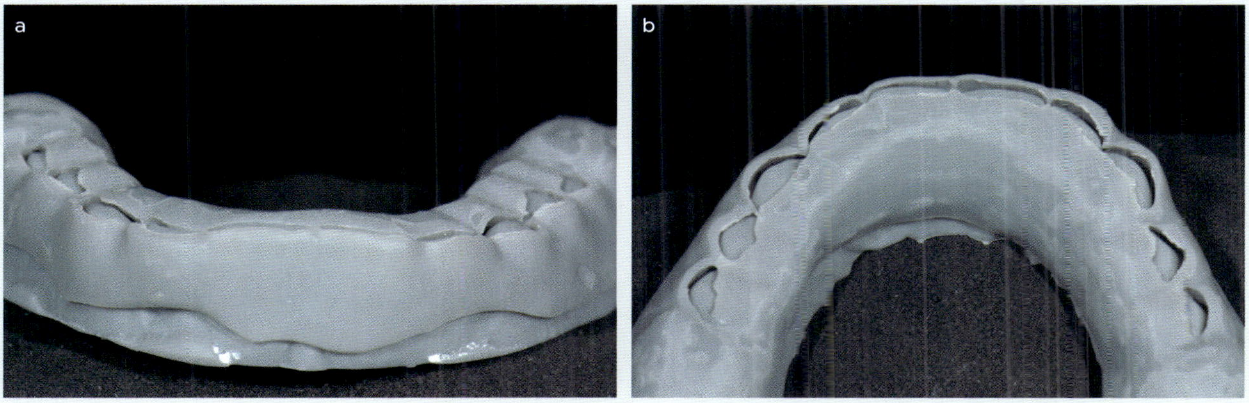

Figure 12 The 3D printed incisal reduction guide.

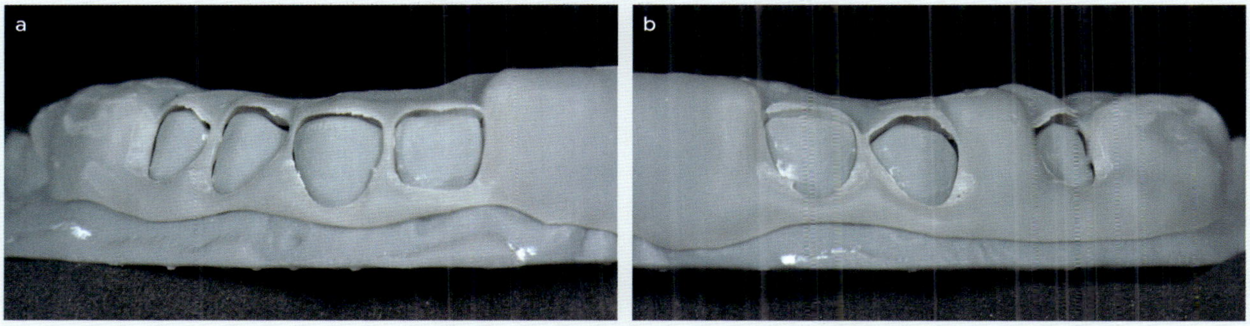

Figure 13 The 3D printed vestibular reduction guide.

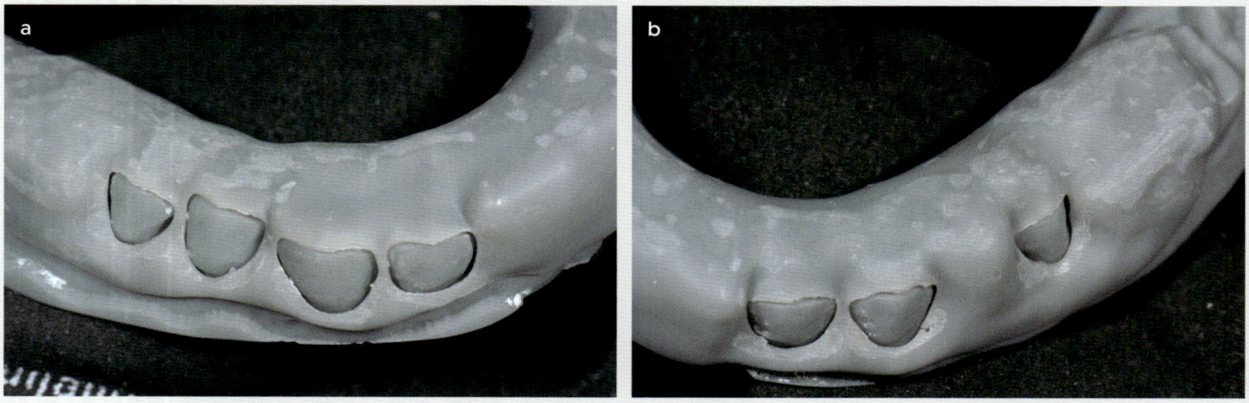

Figure 14 The occlusal view of the vestibular reduction guide on the prepared model demonstrating a single plane of reduction.

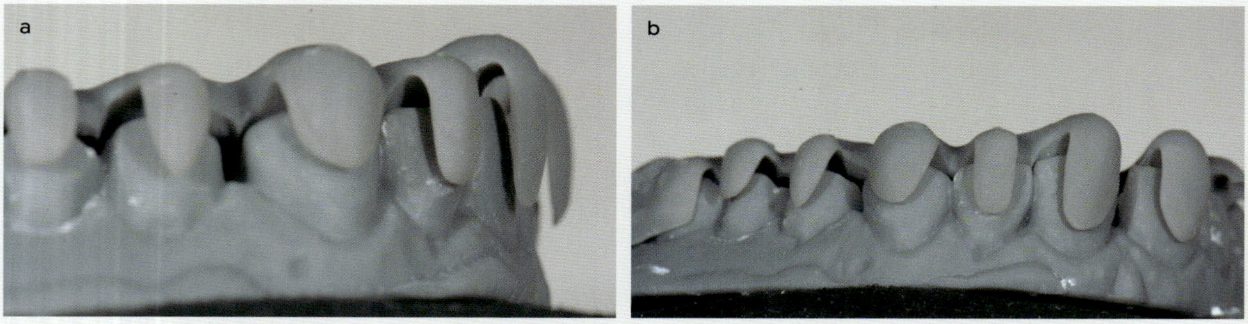

Figure 15 The veneer fit guide on the prepared model.

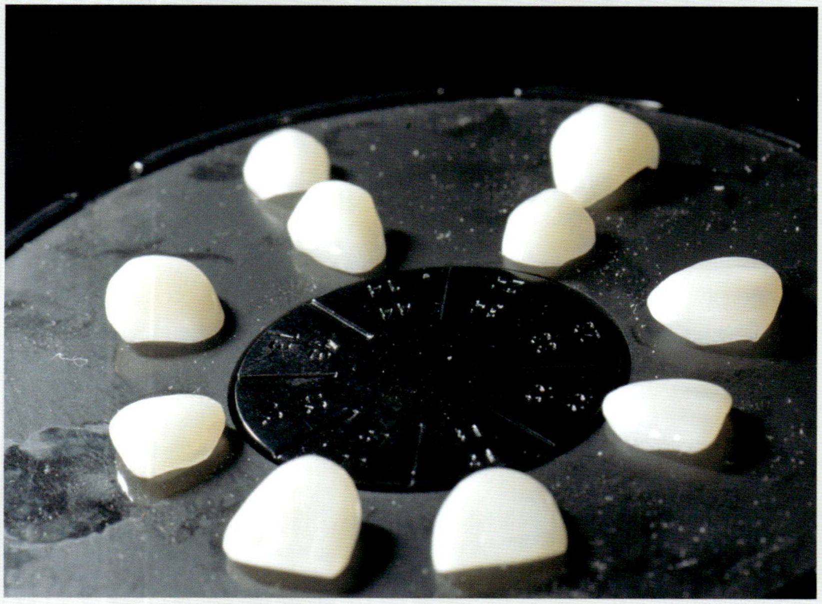

Figure 16 The milled composite veneers.

The incisal reduction guide was placed and any exposed tooth tissue protruding through the guide was marked with a pen (17). This ensured that we had achieved the desired minimum 1.5 mm incisal edge thickness required for material strength in this high-function area. Keeping the bur flat to the guide, any exposed tooth was reduced.

The vestibular reduction guide was then seated and again any tooth protruding from the guide was marked (18). Keeping the bur flat to the plane of the guide, the teeth were flattened in a single plane until no tooth volume was protruding from beyond the margins of the guide. This minimal preparation removed any bulbosities to ensure passive fitting of the final veneers. Following vestibular reduction, there was no removal of cervical enamel and more tooth volume was maintained proximally than with a traditional veneer preparation.

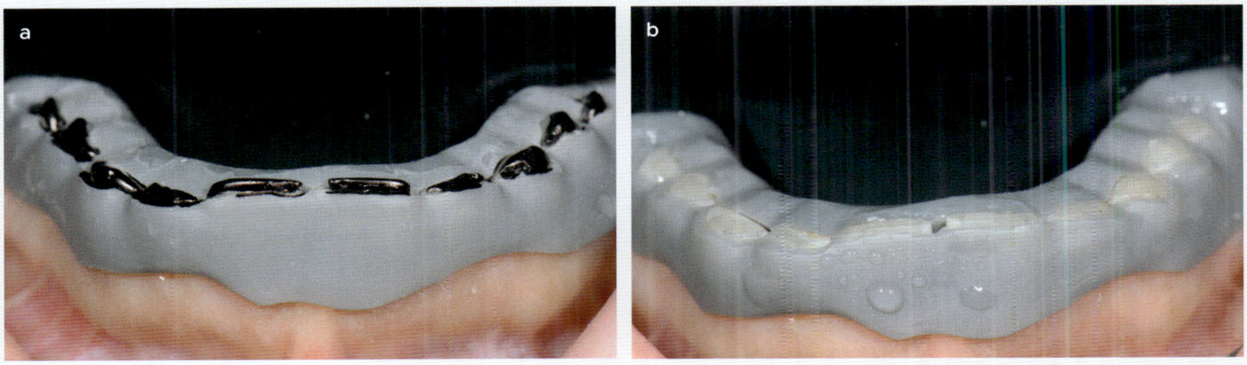

Figure 17 (a) The incisal guide in place with the exposed teeth marked in pen to indicate areas of reduction. (b) Following single-plane preparation, the desired 1.5 mm thickness for material strength is achieved.

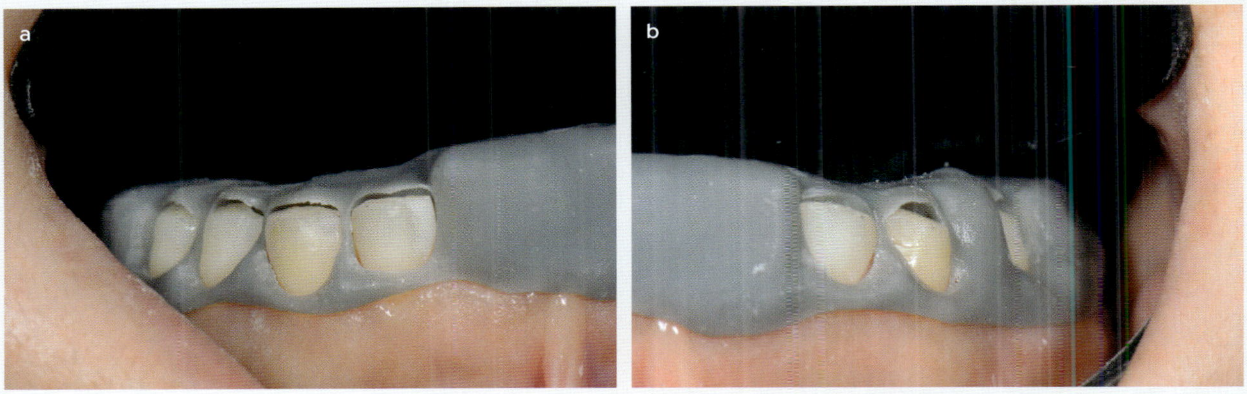

Figure 18 The vestibular reduction guide in place.

Once 2-plane reduction was complete, the contours were smoothed over to remove any sharp angles. The veneers were dry-fitted to assess the margins with the printed fit guide over them to ensure the veneers were accurately seated. The veneers were then pre-treated with adhesive to the fit surface and loaded with flowable composite for cementation. Following the usual steps of sandblasting to remove biofilm and create a micro-mechanical retentive surface, phosphoric acid enamel etching and application of the adhesive, the veneers were placed tooth-by-tooth. The fit guide was then seated allowing the contacts to be cleared with floss and the excess material to be removed without disrupting the position of the veneers.

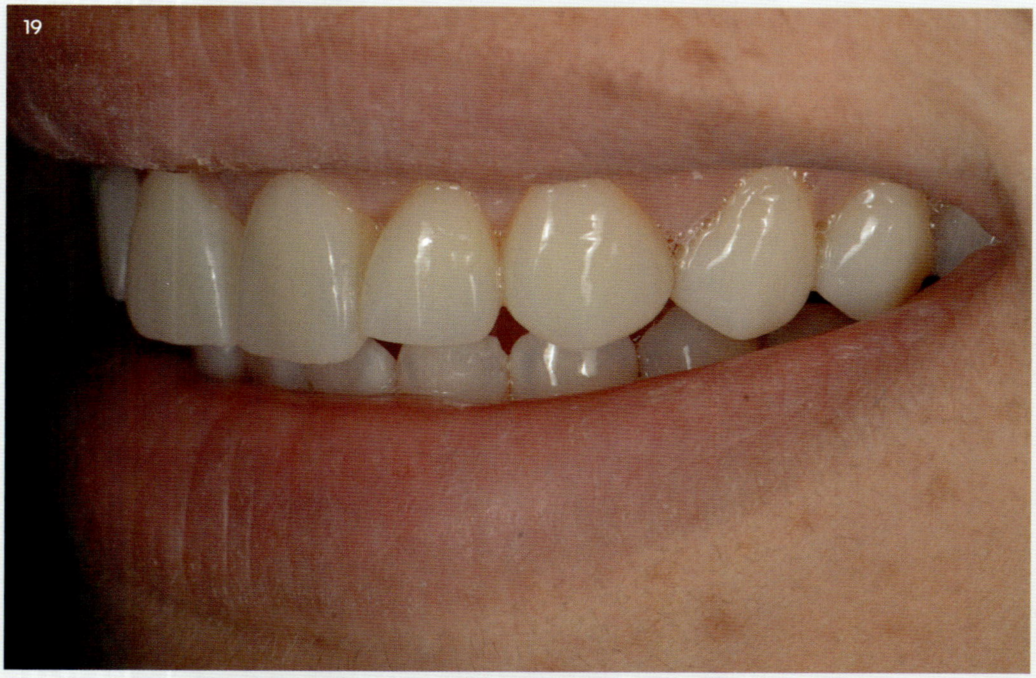

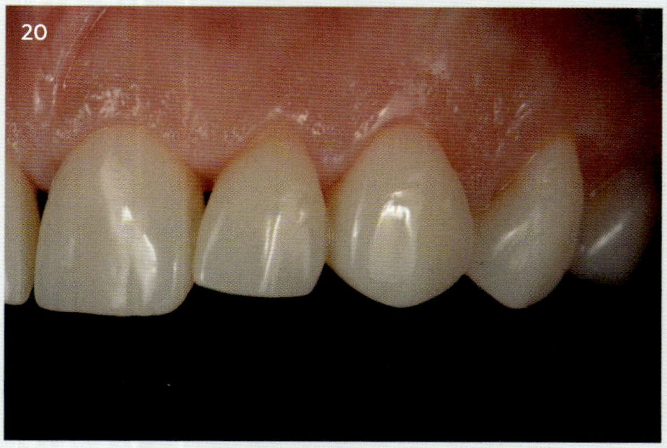

Figure 19 Right lateral smile view of the final smile after polishing.

Figure 20 Right lateral retracted view of the final result.

Figure 21 Left lateral smile view of the final smile after polishing.

Figure 22 Left lateral retracted view of the final result.

Figure 23 Occlusal view demonstrating the additive nature of the veneers.

Following an initial flash cure, the fit guide was removed and the palatal margins were finished before a final cure under glycerin. Once fully cured together, the flowable composite and composite veneer become a single, homogenous strong monolithic restoration. Although the veneer is milled to a knife-edge finish, the final restoration is very strong at the margins once cured and highly resistant to degradation.
The margins around the veneers were then checked for any excess cement and simply cleaned using the LM Excesso instrument and polished (19-23).

21

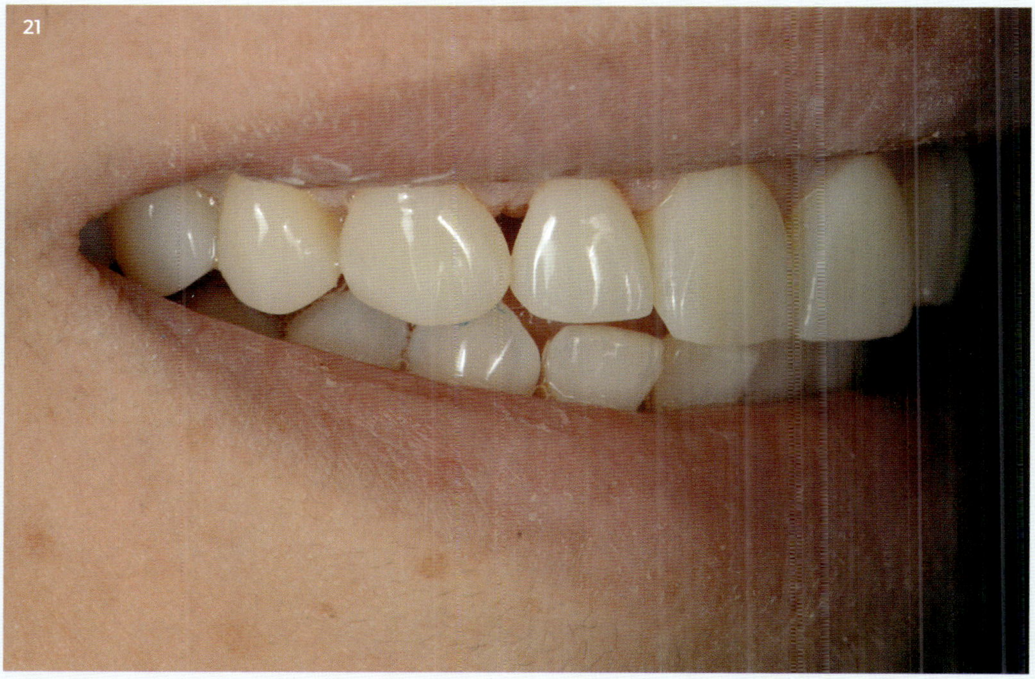

22

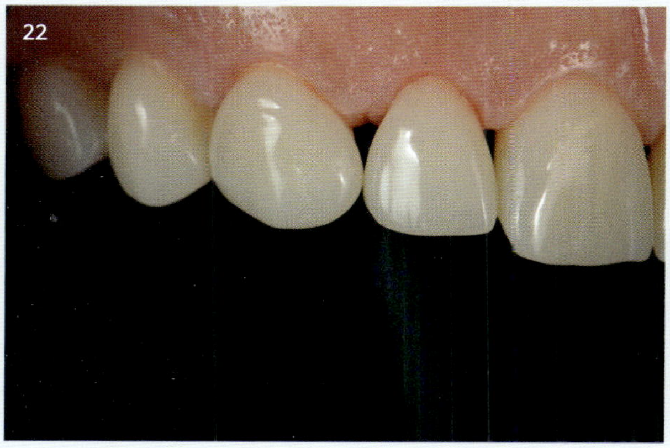

23

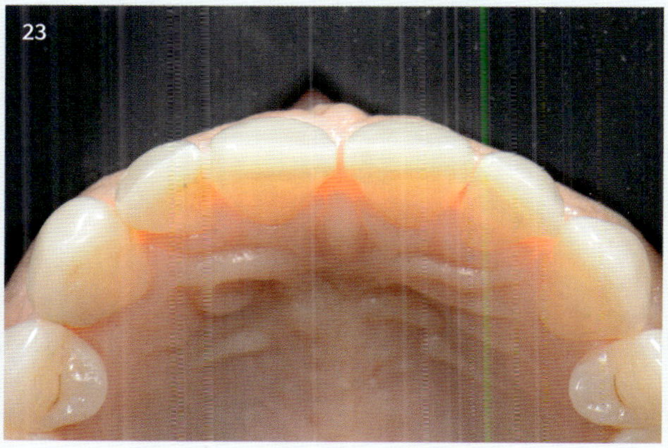

The patient was extremely pleased with the outcome and continues to attend 6-monthly maintenance appointments. At her 2-year follow-up, the veneers have retained their aesthetic appearance, remain intact and the soft tissues exhibit remarkable health (📷 24–26).

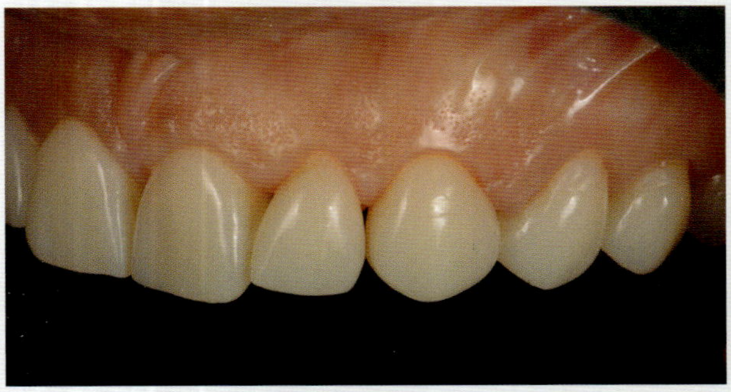

Figure 24 Right lateral view at 2-year follow-up. Note the health of the soft tissue architecture.

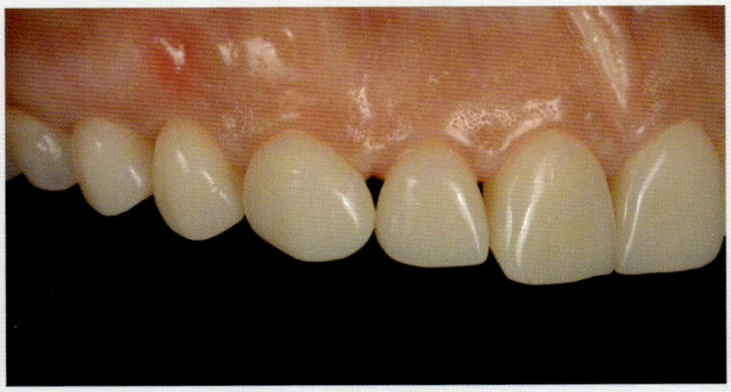

Figure 25 Left lateral view at 2-year follow-up.

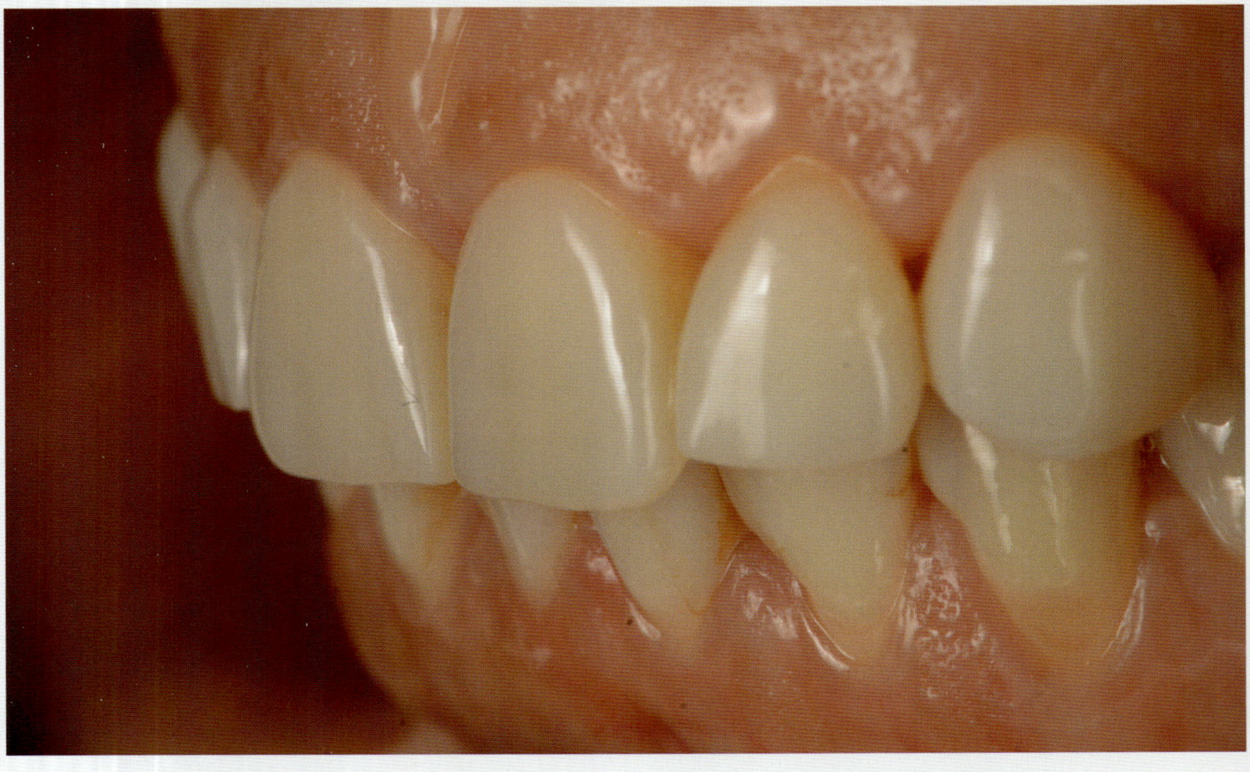

Figure 26 Left lateral retracted view 2-year follow-up.

CONCLUSION

In situations where direct composite proves less than ideal and ceramics are financially out of reach for the patient, it's worth delving into the possibilities offered by indirect composite. The presence of digital dentistry has opened doors to innovative techniques, employing cutting-edge materials for planning and executing smile makeovers with laboratory-milled composite veneers.

Styloso represents a streamlined process, accomplished in a single-visit appointment, significantly reducing chair-time. This approach aided by 3D printed guides, ensures minimal tooth reduction and precision with a simplified and predictable 2-plane reduction technique allowing us to achieve smile makeovers with a ceramic-like finish. Not only is this approach less invasive than traditional veneer preparation, but it also simplifies the process for dentists, reducing stress and complexity and cost.

The forgiving nature of composite materials allows for fast repairs, rejuvenation, adaptation, and or modification at any point, with minimal cost for both the patient and dentist. This provides a significant shift in being able to offer patients flexible and efficient cosmetic dentistry.

SUGGESTED READINGS

- Al-Omiri MK, Lamey PJ, Clifford T. Impact of tooth wear on daily living. *Int J Prosthodont.* 2006;19(6):601-605.
- Bartlett DW, Lussi A, West NX et al. Prevalence of tooth wear on buccal and lingual surfaces and possible risk factors in young European adults. *J Dent.* 2013;41:1007-1013.
- Holbrook WP, Arnadóttir IB, Kay EJ. Prevention. Part 3: prevention of tooth wear. *Br Dent J.* 2003;195(2):75-81.
- Järvinen V, Meurman JH, Hyvärnen H et al. Dental erosion and upper gastrointestinal disorders. *Oral Surg Oral Med Oral Pathol.* 1988;65:298-303.
- Loi I, Di Felice A. Biologically oriented preparation technique (BOPT): a new approach for prosthetic restoration of periodontally healthy teeth. *Eur J Esthet Dent.* 2013;8(1):10-23.
- López-Frías FJ, Castellanos-Cosano L, Martín-González J et al. Clinical measurement of tooth wear: Tooth wear indices. J Clin Exp Dent. 2012;4(1):e43-53.
- Magne P, Douglas WH et al. Additive contour of porcelain veneers: a key element in enamel preservation, adhesion and esthetics for ageing dentition. *J Adhes Dent.* 1999;1(1):81-92.
- Muts EJ, van Pelt H, Edelhoff D et al. Tooth wear: a systematic review of treatment options. *J Prosthet Dent.* 2014;112(4):752-759.
- Spijker AV, Rodriguez JM, Kreulen CM et al. Prevalence of tooth wear in adults. *Int J Prosthodont.* 2009;22:35-42.